Contents

Cen
19/07/04
10:50

This report contains the collective views of an international group of experts and
does not necessarily represent the decisions or the stated policy of the World Health Organization

WHO Technical Report Series

862

HYPERTENSION CONTROL

Report of a
WHO Expert Committee

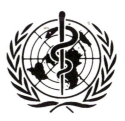

World Health Organization

Geneva 1996

WHO Library Cataloguing in Publication Data

WHO Expert Committee on Hypertension Control
    Hypertension control : report of a WHO expert committee.

    (WHO technical report series ; 862)

    1. Hypertension 2. Risk factors   I. Title II. Series

    ISBN 92 4 120862 7   (NLM Classification: WG 340)
    ISSN 0512-3054

The World Health Organization welcomes requests for permission to reproduce or translate its publications, in part or in full. Applications and enquiries should be addressed to the Office of Publications, World Health Organization, Geneva, Switzerland, which will be glad to provide the latest information on any changes made to the text, plans for new editions, and reprints and translations already available.

Printed in Switzerland
95/10780 – Benteli – 7300

WHO Expert Committee on Hypertension Control

Geneva, 24–31 October 1994

Members

Professor J. P. Chalmers, Department of Medicine, Flinders Medical Centre, Bedford Park, Australia (*Co-Chairman*)

Professor J. G. Fodor, Director of Research, Centre for Prevention and Rehabilitation, University of Ottawa Heart Institute, Ottawa, Ontario, Canada

Professor M. M. Ibrahim, Department of Cardiology, University of Cairo, Cairo, Egypt

Dr C. J. M. Lenfant, Director, National Heart, Lung, and Blood Institute, National Institutes of Health, Bethesda, MD, USA

Professor Liu Li-Sheng, Chief, Department of Cardiology, Fu Wai Hospital, Chinese Academy of Medical Sciences, Beijing, China

Professor J. Menard, Broussais Hospital, Paris, France

Professor B. O. Osuntokun, Professor of Neurology and Dean, Faculty of Medicine, University of Ibadan, Ibadan, Nigeria

Professor K. S. Reddy, Department of Cardiology, Cardiothoracic Centre, All India Institute of Medical Sciences, New Delhi, India (*Rapporteur*)

Professor A. B. Ribeiro, Paulist Medical School, São Paulo, Brazil

Professor L. I. Rilantono, Chief, Department of Cardiology, Faculty of Medicine, Harapan Kita Hospital, University of Indonesia, Slipi-Jakarta, Indonesia

Professor L. Wilhelmsen, Department of Medicine, Ostra Hospital, Gothenburg, Sweden

Professor A. Zanchetti, Director, Centre for Clinical Physiology and Hypertension, Institute of Clinical Medicine and Therapeutics, Ospedale Maggiore, University of Milan, Milan, Italy (*Co-Chairman*)

Representatives of other organizations

International Council of Nurses

Mr T. Ghebrehiwet, Nurse Consultant, International Council of Nurses, Geneva, Switzerland

International Federation of Pharmaceutical Manufacturers Associations

Dr O. Morin, Scientific Executive, International Federation of Pharmaceutical Manufacturers Associations, Geneva, Switzerland

International Society and Federation of Cardiology

Professor J. P. Chalmers (see list of Members)

World Hypertension League

Dr T. Strasser (see Secretariat list)

Secretariat

Dr I. Gyárfás, Chief, Cardiovascular Diseases, WHO, Geneva, Switzerland (*Secretary*)

Dr T. Strasser, Secretary-General, World Hypertension League, Geneva, Switzerland (*Temporary Adviser*)

1. Introduction

A WHO Expert Committee on Hypertension Control met in Geneva from 24 to 31 October 1994. Dr D. E. Barmes, Associate Director, Division of Noncommunicable Diseases, opened the meeting on behalf of the Director-General. He pointed out that hypertension is the commonest cardiovascular disorder, posing a major public health challenge to societies in socioeconomic and epidemiological transition. It is one of the major risk factors for cardiovascular mortality, which accounts for 20–50% of all deaths.

Control of hypertension is a complex, multidimensional process. The objectives are primary prevention, early detection and adequate treatment to prevent complications occurring. Populations and individuals need to be targeted to achieve these objectives. At the population level, changes in lifestyle need to be encouraged using intersectoral collaboration, multidisciplinary approaches, and community involvement and participation; for the individual, hypertension needs to be diagnosed and treated using non-pharmacological and pharmacological methods. Achievement of these objectives also calls for action beyond the health care system, with increased involvement from organizations such as national, regional and international hypertension societies and leagues.

The World Health Organization has been concerned with hypertension since the 1950s. The Expert Committee on Cardiovascular Diseases and Hypertension, convened in October 1958 in Geneva, gave special consideration to the classification and criteria for the diagnosis of hypertension (1). A subsequent Expert Committee met in Geneva in October 1961. It described the stages of hypertension but its recommendations were limited to therapeutic remedies directed against the progressive effect of diseases (secondary prevention) (2). A third Expert Committee met in Geneva in March 1978 and dealt with the epidemiology, prevention and control of hypertension (3).

The present Expert Committee met to review the epidemiology of hypertension in order to increase awareness particularly in developing countries, to analyse the experience gained by community control programmes, and to discuss options for prevention and management strategies.

The main aims of this report are to establish the control of hypertension as part of programmes to reduce total cardiovascular risk, to focus attention on the population approach to primary prevention of hypertension, and to summarize appropriate clinical approaches and management options for the hypertensive patient. The report also emphasizes the importance of systolic blood pressure in defining and managing high blood pressure and extends recommendations for the control of hypertension to the elderly. The consideration of effectiveness and cost with respect to prevention and management is introduced to assist the selection of optimal strategies in different socioeconomic settings.

The report offers guidelines to decision-makers in public health, to managers of hypertension control programmes, and to physicians involved in the clinical management of the hypertensive patient, and recommends that the control of hypertension should be an integral part of national health care systems.

2. Definition and classification of hypertension

2.1 Definition

2.1.1 *Operational definition of hypertension*

Definition of hypertension is difficult and, by necessity, arbitrary. Sir George Pickering first formulated the concept that blood pressure in a population is distributed continuously as a bell-shaped curve with no real separation between "normotension" and "hypertension" (*4*). There is also a direct relation between cardiovascular risk and blood pressure: the higher the blood pressure, the higher the risk of both stroke and coronary events (*5*). As a consequence, the dividing line between "normotension" and "hypertension" can be defined only in an operational way: Evans & Rose (*6*) defined it as that level of blood pressure at which detection and treatment do more good than harm. This level can be determined only by intervention trials demonstrating benefits from blood pressure reduction.

As intervention trials have included only adult subjects aged 18 years or older, the following sections on definition and classification of hypertension refer to adults. The problem of hypertension in children is discussed separately in section 7.2.1.

2.1.2 *Definition of hypertension based on diastolic and/or systolic blood pressure*

High diastolic blood pressure has commonly been used to define hypertension. This arbitrary choice was based on the fact that diastolic blood pressure was used as the criterion for inclusion in most randomized therapeutic trials, including those on mild hypertension. There is, however, mounting evidence that systolic values should also be taken into account in defining, as well as managing, hypertension (*7*). Indeed, cardiovascular risk is as strongly associated with systolic as with diastolic values, with no evidence of a threshold below which a decrease in systolic pressure does not reduce risk. Furthermore, some of the intervention trials on mild hypertension indicate that cardiovascular events more closely correlate with systolic than with diastolic values achieved by treatment (*8*).

Hypertension should therefore be defined using both diastolic and systolic blood pressures. Patients whose resting values of diastolic blood pressure remain persistently at or above 90 mmHg (12.0 kPa) after repeated measurements are at increased risk of cardiovascular morbidity and mortality, and lowering of diastolic blood pressure values of between 90 and 105 mmHg (12.0 and 14.0 kPa) has been clearly shown to reduce the risk of stroke by 35-40% and of coronary events by about 15-20% (9). From epidemiological data on incidence of strokes and coronary events, the range of systolic blood pressures corresponding to diastolic values of 90-105 mmHg (12.0-14.0 kPa) is approximately 140-180 mmHg (18.7-24.0 kPa) (7), and intervention trials have shown treatment benefits when systolic blood pressure values of, or greater than, 160 mmHg (21.3 kPa) are lowered (10, 11).

The current definition of hypertension is therefore a level of systolic blood pressure of 140 mmHg (18.7 kPa) or above, or a level of diastolic blood pressure of 90 mmHg (12.0 kPa) or above. However, as blood pressure is quite variable, before labelling a patient as hypertensive and deciding to initiate treatment, it is necessary to confirm raised levels of blood pressure by repeated measurements over periods of several weeks. Whenever values in the mild or borderline hypertension range (see below) are found, confirmatory measurements should be extended over 3-6 months. Shorter observation periods are required in patients with more marked elevations of blood pressure or in those with complications (12, 13).

2.1.3 Hypertension and total cardiovascular risk

Hypertension is one of several risk factors for cardiovascular disease. The known factors are listed in Table 1. When the level of blood pressure is only slightly above the threshold for definition of hypertension, the presence of one or more of these factors may be a more important determinant of the patient's risk, especially of a coronary event, than the increase in blood pressure.

Since the absolute benefits of treatment for hypertension will be determined by the absolute risk of cardiovascular disease (i.e. greater benefits for those at higher risk), each of these factors should be assessed before deciding on treatment.

The absolute risk of serious cardiovascular disease varies greatly among individuals with mild hypertension. At one extreme, in elderly patients with a history of cardiovascular disease, at least 3-5 in 100 will suffer a further serious event each year (10, 11, 14, 15). At the other extreme, in young patients with no other risk factors, fewer than 1 in 1000 will suffer a serious event each year (8, 16). Although treatment for hypertension will reduce risk in both of these patient populations, it may take some decades for clinical benefits to become apparent in young patients at low initial risk.

The absolute risk of cardiovascular disease in mild hypertension may also vary substantially from one geographical region to another. Some of the regional variation in the risk of stroke and coronary events may be accounted for by regional differences in the prevalence of the risk factors

Table 1
Risk factors for cardiovascular disease

Age[a]

Sex[a]

Family history of premature cardiovascular disease[a]

Raised systolic blood pressure

Raised diastolic blood pressure

Smoking

Raised serum levels of total and low-density lipoprotein-cholesterol

Reduced serum levels of high-density lipoprotein-cholesterol

Left ventricular hypertrophy

Previous cardiovascular events[a]

Previous cerebrovascular events[a]

Diabetes

Renal disease

Micro-albuminuria

Obesity

Sedentary lifestyle

---

[a] Not modifiable.
Source: reference *12*.

listed in Table 1. However, other evidence indicates that there are some regional differences that cannot be accounted for by differences in established risk factors. Of particular note are the high rates of stroke in China and the Russian Federation. In these populations stroke incidence is four times that in the United States of America and western Europe, but the average blood pressure is only slightly higher (*12*). For this reason, the treatment of mild hypertension in these populations may be particularly beneficial.

2.2 Blood pressure measurement

2.2.1 *Devices and methods*

Blood pressure is generally measured indirectly using a mercury sphygmomanometer and the auscultatory method.

Before the measurement is taken, the patient should be seated for several minutes in a quiet room in a chair that supports the back comfortably. The arm muscles should be relaxed and the forearm supported with the cubital fossa at heart level (fourth intercostal space). Blood pressure may also be measured with the subject supine or standing providing that the arm is supported at heart level. The patient should avoid wearing anything with tight sleeves. A cuff of suitable size is applied evenly to the exposed upper arm. A cuff for adults must have a bladder 13-15 cm wide and 30-35 cm long so as to encircle the average arm; the standard cuff available in many countries may be too small. Larger cuffs are needed for fat arms and smaller cuffs for children. The cuff is rapidly inflated until the manometer reading is about 30 mmHg (4.0 kPa) above the level at which the pulse disappears, and then slowly deflated at approximately 2 mmHg/s (0.3 kPa/s). During this time the Korotkoff sounds are monitored using a stethoscope placed over the brachial artery.

The pressure at which the sounds are first heard is the systolic blood pressure (SBP). The diastolic blood pressure (DBP) is the pressure at the point when the sounds disappear (phase V). Most major studies have used this point, i.e. disappearance of sounds, for identifying DBP; the use of muffling sounds (phase IV) gives significantly higher DBP values, and is to be avoided. Systolic and diastolic blood pressure should be measured at least twice over a period of no less than three minutes; both should be recorded and the mean value for each calculated. It is also recommended that, on the first visit, the patient's blood pressure is measured on both arms and in the sitting and standing position. Blood pressure should regularly be measured with the patient standing if postural hypotension is suspected, and in the elderly in whom this condition may be more common.

Some devices for measuring blood pressure use an aneroid instead of a mercury manometer. Aneroid manometers are subject to inaccuracies and, whenever used, should be calibrated and regularly checked against a mercury column. Automatic and semi-automatic devices with a digital display should also be calibrated and periodically checked. Some of these devices measure blood pressure by an oscillometric method rather than by monitoring Korotkoff sounds; blood pressure values measured by the two different methods (auscultatory versus oscillometric) should be compared to check accuracy.

Some automatic machines have been adapted for measurement of blood pressure at pre-set intervals over several hours in the ambulatory patient. These devices too should be carefully checked, preferably in ambulatory conditions.

Beat-to-beat blood pressure measurement is feasible by direct intra-arterial monitoring in the ambulatory patient, but should be reserved for particular research conditions. Non-invasive beat-to-beat blood pressure monitoring is also possible using a device placed on the finger, with the patient seated or supine. A portable device is being developed to obtain ambulatory readings.

2.2.2 *Clinic or office blood pressure measurement*

Blood pressure is usually measured in an outpatient clinic, in a physician's office or at the patient's bedside by a mercury sphygmomanometer using the auscultatory method, according to the guidelines given in section 2.2.1. These values are usually referred to as "clinic" or "office" blood pressures, and are those measured in all intervention trials by which the benefits of antihypertensive therapy and therefore the current operational definition of hypertension have been established.

2.2.3 *Home and ambulatory blood pressure measurements*

Semi-automatic and automatic devices and, sometimes, aneroid or mercury sphygmomanometers are increasingly being used at home to measure blood pressure by the patients themselves (self-measurement) or by a relative. This has the undoubted advantage of providing more numerous measurements and measurements taken in a more relaxed setting than the physician's office or outpatient clinic (*12*). Patients or their relatives should receive appropriate instructions in order to ensure reliable measurements.

Monitoring ambulatory blood pressure is an interesting research technique used to investigate blood pressure variability, behavioural influences on arterial pressure and the effects of antihypertensive therapy over time (*12*). It is also used, as are home blood-pressure readings, to supplement information for diagnostic and therapeutic decisions. While these procedures are of potential clinical interest, several issues need to be resolved before their widespread use can be recommended (*17*). Home and ambulatory blood pressure values cannot be equated to readings taken by the conventional method in the clinic by physicians or nurses. Indeed, a recent population survey (the Pamela Study) has shown that both home blood pressure and ambulatory blood pressure values averaged over 24 hours are several mmHg lower than values measured in the clinic; this difference becomes greater with advancing age and at higher clinic blood pressures (*18*).

The causes of these differences between blood pressure values measured in various settings and by various methods are not clear. The presence of a physician and, to a lesser degree, of a nurse can cause some emotional elevation of blood pressure ("white-coat effect") (*19*). However, the use of the term "white-coat hypertension" when a subject's blood pressure is in the hypertensive range in the clinic and is definitely lower at home or under ambulatory conditions is questionable and should be discouraged. In particular, it should be remembered that prospective studies to identify prognostically valuable standards for home or ambulatory blood pressures have not been conducted. There is also no proof that people with so-called white-coat hypertension have "emotional" hypertension, are at no increased risk, and do not deserve treatment. Indeed it has been suggested that these subjects (who may be more properly described as having isolated "clinic" hypertension) may have a higher cardiovascular risk than normotensive subjects (20). The phenomenon of isolated "clinic" hypertension has clinical relevance and should be investigated in depth. For now, physicians should remember that home and ambulatory blood pressure readings are on average several mmHg lower than clinic values, particularly in the elderly (18), and set thresholds for hypertension and target blood pressure for treatment at a lower level to avoid underdiagnosis and undertreatment (12).

2.3 Classification of hypertension

Classification of hypertension based on epidemiological, observational and interventional data, and taking into consideration associated risk factors and development of hypertension-related organ damage, provides an easy and reliable method of assessing risk and the most appropriate treatment for each patient. With the obvious warning that all classifications of hypertension are based on arbitrary choices, arterial hypertension may be classified in three ways by: blood pressure, extent of damage to the organs and etiology.

2.3.1 *Blood pressure*

The risk associated with raised blood pressure increases progressively (4), and the dividing line between "normotension" and "hypertension" is arbitrary. However, the considerations made in the preceding sections allow an operational classification of hypertension to be made. This classification is illustrated in Table 2 as a practical guide to management.

In this classification the terms "mild", "moderate" and "severe" hypertension have been retained because of their common use in the

Table 2
Classification of hypertension by blood pressure level

	Systolic and diastolic blood pressure (SBP and DBP), mmHg (kPa)	
Normotension	<140 (<18.7) SBP and	<90 (<12.0) DBP
Mild hypertension	140–180 (18.7–24.0) SBP or	90–105 (12.0–14.0) DBP
Subgroup: borderline	140–160 (18.7–21.3) SBP or	90–95 (12.0–12.7) DBP
Moderate and severe hypertension[a]	>180 (>24.0) SBP or	>105 (>14.0) DBP
Isolated systolic hypertension	>140 (>18.7) SBP and	<90 (<12.0) DBP
Subgroup: borderline	140–160 (18.7–21.3) SBP and	<90 (<12.0) DBP

[a] Risk to be indicated by reporting the actual values of SBP and DBP.
Source: reference 12.

clinical setting. It should be emphasized that, as currently used, these terms do not refer to the severity of the overall clinical condition, but simply to the extent of the blood pressure elevation (*12*). As mentioned in section 2.1.3, the severity of the clinical condition also depends on the overall cardiovascular risk of the patient, which is influenced by concomitant risk factors such as age, sex, smoking habits and level of plasma lipids. Associated organ damage is a particularly important risk factor and may be a better indicator of the severity of the clinical condition than blood pressure (section 2.3.2).

The term "mild" hypertension is used to refer to individuals with either DBP of 90-105 mmHg (12.0-14.0 kPa) or SBP of 140-180 mmHg (18.7-24.0 kPa). The term "borderline" hypertension is used in the subgroup of mild hypertensive subjects with DBP of 90-95 mmHg (12.0-12.7 kPa) or SBP of 140-160 mmHg (18.7-21.3 kPa). The term "mild" is used to describe blood pressure that is mildly elevated, but it does not always imply that the absolute risk of cardiovascular disease is only slightly elevated. For instance, in an individual at high risk of stroke or myocardial infarction, mild hypertension may considerably aggravate this risk, and reducing the blood pressure is likely to confer large benefits. The same considerations apply to patients with diabetic nephropathy. Furthermore, the high prevalence of mild hypertension results in a correspondingly high health burden for populations (*12*).

The terms "moderate" and "severe" hypertension are used to indicate progressively more marked elevations of systolic and diastolic blood pressure, and do not imply a moderate or severe overall risk. It is suggested that, outside the "mild" hypertension range, the risk associated with blood pressure is better indicated by reporting the actual values of systolic and diastolic blood pressure.

"Isolated systolic hypertension" is a comprehensive term indicating all patients with SBP greater than 140 mmHg (18.7 kPa) and DBP less than 90 mmHg (12.0 kPa). The benefits of treating isolated systolic hypertension have so far been shown only for patients with SBP levels or, of greater than, 160 mmHg (21.3 kPa). Patients with SBP of 140-160 mmHg (18.7-21.3 kPa) and DBP lower than 90 mmHg (12.0 kPa) should be classified as having "borderline" isolated systolic hypertension (*12*).

Classifying patients with DBP of 85-89 mmHg (11.3-11.9 kPa) or SBP of 130-139 mmHg (17.3-18.5 kPa) as "high normal" (*17*) does not appear to be justified at present, and carries the risk of labelling a very large number.

2.3.2 *Organ damage*

Although the extent of organ damage often correlates with the level of blood pressure, it is not always the case. In addition the rate of progression of organ damage varies from one individual to another depending on many influences, most of which are incompletely understood. Therefore, blood pressure and organ impairment should be evaluated separately, since markedly high pressures may be seen without organ damage and, conversely, organ damage may be present with only moderate elevation of blood pressure. The presence of signs of organ damage confers an increased cardiovascular risk to any level of blood pressure. The classification of hypertension by extent of organ damage (Table 3) uses stages to indicate progression of the severity of disease with time.

Table 3
Classification of hypertension by extent of organ damage

Stage I	No manifestations of organic change
Stage II	At least one of the following manifestations of organ involvement
	Left ventricular hypertrophy (detected by radiogram, electrocardiogram, echocardiogram)
	Generalized and focal narrowing of the retinal arteries
	Micro-albuminuria, proteinuria and/or slight elevation of the plasma creatinine concentration (1.2–2.0 mg/dl)
	Ultrasound or radiological evidence of atherosclerotic plaque (in the aorta or carotid, iliac or femoral arteries)
Stage III	Both symptoms and signs have appeared as a result of organ damage. These include

	Heart
	    Angina pectoris
	    Myocardial infarction
	    Heart failure

	Brain
	    Stroke
	    Transient ischaemic attack
	    Hypertensive encephalopathy
	    Vascular dementia

	Optic fundi Retinal haemorrhages and exudates with or without papilloedema (these features are pathognomonic of the malignant or accelerated phase – see section 6)

	Kidney
	    Plasma creatinine concentration >2.0 mg/dl
	    Renal failure

	Vessel
	    Dissecting aneurysm
	    Symptomatic arterial occlusive disease

Source: WHO Expert Committee on Arterial Hypertension (3) and the 1993 guidelines for the management of mild hypertension (12).

Precise staging of hypertension by extent of organ damage will depend on diagnostic procedures, some of them costly or uncomfortable for the patient. It is not implied that all these procedures should be carried out in each patient, as subsequently discussed in section 7.1 on diagnosis of the hypertensive patient.

2.3.3 *Etiology*

In over 95% of patients with hypertension no specific cause can be identified. These patients are diagnosed as having primary hypertension. The small minority of patients in whom a specific cause can be identified are diagnosed as having secondary hypertension. A more detailed discussion of secondary hypertension is given in section 5.

3. Epidemiology of high blood pressure

3.1 High blood pressure as a risk factor

Epidemiological studies have consistently identified an important and independent link between high blood pressure and various disorders, especially coronary heart disease, stroke, congestive heart failure and impaired renal function.

Quantitative estimates based on pooled data from nine prospective observational studies, corrected for regression dilution bias, indicate that subjects with DBP of 105 mmHg (14.0 kPa) have a tenfold increase in the risk of stroke and a fivefold increase in risk of coronary events compared with those with DBP of 76 mmHg (10.1 kPa). These findings suggest that prolonged reductions in usual DBP of 5, 7.5 and 10 mmHg (0.67, 1.0 and 1.33 kPa) are respectively associated with at least 34%, 46% and 56% less stroke and at least 21%, 29% and 37% fewer coronary events (5).

While both systolic and diastolic blood pressures have been consistently identified as independent risk factors, SBP has been associated with a higher relative risk of coronary heart disease, stroke, congestive heart failure, renal disease and general mortality for a similar range of blood pressure. In the follow up of the Multiple Risk Factor Intervention Trial (MRFIT) carried out by Stamler, Stamler & Neaton (*21*), relative risk of coronary events increased progressively from 1.0 in those with an optimum SBP of less than 120 mmHg (16.0 kPa) and DBP less than 80 mmHg (10.7 kPa) to 3.23 in those with an isolated increase of DBP to, or greater than, 100 mmHg (13.3 kPa); 4.19 in those with an isolated increase of SBP to, or greater than, 160 mmHg (21.3 kPa); and 4.57 in those with a combined increase of SBP to, or greater than, 160 mmHg (21.3 kPa) and of DBP to, or greater than, 100 mmHg (13.3 kPa).

In a 34-year follow up of the Framingham Heart Study cohort, the risk of congestive heart failure was 2-4 times higher for those in the highest quintile of blood pressure than for those in the lowest (22). In the MRFIT screening cohort (21), followed for 15.3 years, the covariate-adjusted risk of end-stage renal disease for a 10 mmHg (1.33 kPa) rise in SBP above baseline was 1.65 (95% confidence interval 1.57–1.76).

The relation between blood pressure and cardiovascular disease has been found to be consistent in large observational studies conducted in both sexes and in varied populations. The risk rises progressively with increased blood pressure, with no evidence of a threshold for risk or a J-shaped relationship (23). This continuum of risk makes the definition of the cut-off point for hypertension arbitrary.

Although high blood pressure is independently associated with an increased risk of cardiovascular events, the risk is substantially increased by the presence and levels of other risk factors like smoking, elevated serum cholesterol and diabetes (Fig. 1). As a consequence, equal blood pressure levels carry different risks when associated with different combinations of risk factors. Assessing the total risk of cardiovascular disease has important implications for defining intervention thresholds in individuals with high blood pressure (24).

When comparing the prevalence of hypertension in different populations, the variability contributed by differing survey methodologies and by different cut-off points needs to be considered. The recognition of blood pressure as a continuous biological variable, however, makes it possible to compare the distribution in different populations irrespective of the cut-off points used to define hypertension. This is validated by the observation that mean blood pressure levels in different populations are a good indication of the prevalence of hypertension. Therefore, as the distribution of blood pressure in a population shifts to the left, the prevalence of hypertension decreases, irrespective of the cut-off point used to define it.

The study of the distribution of blood pressure is also valuable in highlighting the need to lower blood pressure across the whole population rather than targeting those at highest risk. Although the relative risk is highest in those identified as having severely elevated blood pressure (whichever classification system is used), there are considerably fewer people in this category than in the group identified as having mildly elevated blood pressure. Whatever the cut-off points, the population with raised blood pressure constitutes a risk pyramid, with the largest number at the base where the relative risk is elevated but not high, and the smallest number at the top where the relative risk is the greatest. Therefore the greatest absolute number of complications attributable to high blood pressure occurs at the base of the pyramid, i.e. in those categorized as having mildly elevated blood pressure. In the follow up of people screened for MRFIT, the excess deaths from coronary heart disease attributable to high blood pressure were 42.9%, 16.9% and 7.2% in the three SBP categories of 140–159 mmHg (18.7–21.2 kPa), 160–179 mmHg (21.3–23 kPa) and ≥180 mmHg (≥24.0 kPa), respectively (Fig. 2).

Figure 1
The importance of risk-factor combinations, illustrated by the six-year risk of myocardial infarction at various levels of SBP and serum cholesterol in smokers and non-smokers

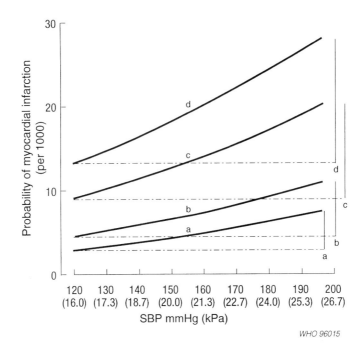

WHO 96015

The vertical axis gives the probability of myocardial infarction occurring in the next 6 years per 1000 men with a given SBP.

Curve a: risk in the absence of smoking and elevated serum cholesterol.
Curve b: risk in smokers.
Curve c: risk with elevated serum cholesterol.
Curve d: risk with smoking and elevated serum cholesterol.

The vertical bars a–d show how the increment in the risk of myocardial infarction associated with a given SBP elevation depends on the various "constellations" (combinations) of risk factors. The *ratios* of the lengths of the bars provide a measure of the risk due to a particular risk-factor constellation.

Adapted, with permission, from Strasser (*24*).

This highlights the need to reduce blood pressure in people with "mild" hypertension in order to achieve substantial reductions in complications in the community as a whole, while protecting individuals at highest risk of developing complications associated with severely elevated blood pressure.

Figure 2

The risk pyramid for blood pressure and coronary heart disease (CHD): baseline SBP and CHD death rates for men screened in MRFIT

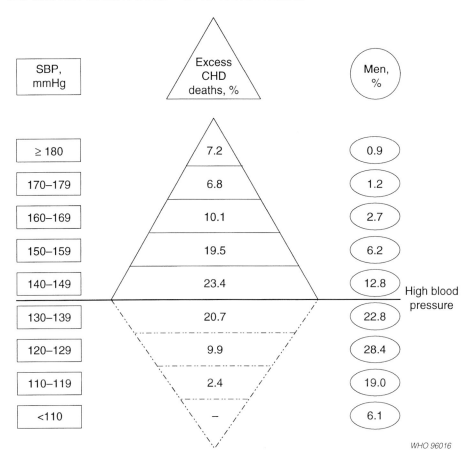

Adapted with permission from Stamler J, Stamler R, Neaton JD. Blood pressure, systolic and diastolic, and cardiovascular risks: US population data. *Archives of internal medicine,* 1993, 153:598-615; copyright 1993, American Medical Association.

3.2 Factors influencing blood pressure

3.2.1 *Age*

Cross-sectional surveys, as well as prospective observational cohort studies, have consistently demonstrated a positive relation between age and blood pressure in most populations with diverse geographical, cultural and socioeconomic characteristics (*23*).

In most western populations, SBP tends to rise progressively throughout childhood, adolescence and adulthood to attain an average value of 140 mmHg (18.7 kPa) by the seventh or eighth decade. DBP also tends to increase with age but at a slower rate than for SBP, and the average value tends to remain flat or decline after the fifth decade. This leads to an increase in pulse pressure, with isolated increases of SBP becoming more common with advancing age.

However, in some isolated populations (e.g. Yanamamo Indians in Brazil and Kenyan nomads) this age-related rise of blood pressure is not evident. This is especially true of populations with low salt intakes (*23, 25*). It has also been observed that unacculturated societies acquire a predisposition to age-related increases in blood pressure when they adopt a western lifestyle, indicating an environmental influence (especially the effects of dietary changes). Thus, there is a reason to believe that age-related rise of blood pressure is neither an inevitable nor a normal biological accompaniment of the aging process.

3.2.2 *Sex*

Early in life there is little evidence of a difference in blood pressure between the sexes. Beginning at adolescence, however, men tend to display a higher average level. This difference is most evident in young and middle-aged adults. Late in life the difference narrows and the pattern may even be reversed (*23*). While this change late in life is partly accounted for by the higher premature death rates of middle-aged men with high blood pressure, post-menopausal changes in women also may be contributory. Studies are in progress to evaluate whether estrogen supplementation protects against the late relative rise of blood pressure in women.

3.2.3 *Ethnicity*

Population studies have consistently revealed higher blood pressure levels in black communities than other ethnic groups (*23*). Ethnicity may influence the relation of age and blood pressure, as indicated by the progressive age-related trend in higher blood pressures in black Americans of African origin than in whites. Average differences in blood pressure between the two groups vary from slightly less than 5 mmHg (0.67 kPa) during the second decade of life to nearly 20 mmHg (2.67 kPa) during the sixth. Black Americans of African origin have also been demonstrated to have higher blood pressure levels than black Africans, suggesting the environmental augmentation of an ethnic predisposition. The role of ethnicity, independent of environmental factors, needs to be clarified in other ethnic groups in countries with ethnic diversity.

3.2.4 *Socioeconomic status*

In countries that are in the post-transitional stage of economic and epidemiological change, consistently higher levels of blood pressure and a higher prevalence of hypertension have been noted in lower socioeconomic groups. This inverse relation has been noted with levels of education, income and occupation. However, in societies that are transitional or pre-transitional, higher levels of blood pressure and a higher prevalence of hypertension have been noted in upper socioeconomic groups. This probably represents the initial stage of the epidemic of cardiovascular disease. Experience in most societies has revealed a reversal of the social groups affected as the epidemic advances.

3.3 The prevalence of hypertension

Estimates of the prevalence of hypertension depend on the cut-off point by which it is defined. Since there is a direct relation between blood pressure and risk of complications, the decision is arbitrary as to who is sick and who is healthy. However, population surveys providing estimates of the prevalence of hypertension are a useful indication of the magnitude of the problem. When assessing the prevalence of hypertension, those people who are being treated for hypertension at the time of the survey should be included, regardless of their actual blood pressure level.

There is a large body of literature estimating the prevalence of hypertension in various parts of the world (26–33). These estimates can be compared only with the utmost caution because differences in the definition of hypertension, measurement methods used, observers and age structures of populations may not have been standardized. Furthermore, some estimates are based on studies using casual one-off blood pressure readings which tend to overestimate the prevalence of hypertension since a proportion of people with a high reading will return to the normotensive range. While such casual blood pressure readings partly predict future risk, it is recommended that prevalence estimates be based on surveys in which measurements are repeated, at least in representative sub-samples. This will provide more accurate estimates of the problem of clinically relevant hypertension and avoid the problems of false labelling.

Despite these limitations, prevalence estimates from several parts of the world indicate that high blood pressure is an important public health problem of global dimensions. When threshold values are taken as 160 mmHg (21.3 kPa) SBP and 95 mmHg (12.7 kPa) DBP, the prevalence of hypertension is reported to be between 10% and 20% in several adult populations. If threshold values of 140 mmHg (18.7 kPa) SBP and 90 mmHg (12.0 kPa) DBP were used, the prevalence estimates would be even higher. Prevalence of hypertension increases with age and shows a relative male preponderance below the age of 50 years. Some geographical diversity has been noted, with industrial countries reporting higher prevalence rates than most developing countries. Differences between urban and rural areas have been reported in some developing countries, with higher prevalence estimates in urban communities. Ethnic differences, such as higher prevalence rates in blacks than whites, have been reported from some countries.

Within regions, and even within individual countries, it would be useful to obtain disaggregated data on the prevalence of hypertension in various ethnic and geographical groups in order to facilitate control and monitoring programmes.

3.4 Risk factors and predictors of high blood pressure

Changes in blood pressure are manifestations of an altered interplay between the neurohumoral, metabolic and haemodynamic mechanisms that regulate basal levels and responses to various stimuli. It is possible to identify the aberrations in these mechanisms that characterize elevated blood pressure, but elucidation of the risk factors that contribute to them requires the following criteria of causality to be met: strength and consistency of association, the cause preceding the effect, a dose-response relationship, compatibility with current biological knowledge, epidemiological validity independent of confounding factors and, whenever possible, experimental evidence in humans.

A search for risk factors in people with established high blood pressure would be too late in the natural history of the disease because of post-morbid modifications caused by disease and interventions. Furthermore, cause and effect cannot be established in such a setting. The major epidemiological evidence must come from observational studies of prospective cohorts and intervention trials, with ecological studies of interpopulation differences and time trends generating hypotheses or providing supplementary evidence.

3.4.1 *Heredity*

A family history of elevated blood pressure is one of the strongest risk factors for future development of hypertension in individuals. The blood pressures of first-order adult relatives (parents, siblings), corrected for age and sex, have been shown to aggregate at all levels of blood pressure, with a regression coefficient of 0.2–0.3 (*34*).

Long-term longitudinal studies of blood pressure in adult populations have shown that individuals tend to retain their blood pressure rank relative to others. Further studies have shown that this "tracking phenomenon" can be followed from early childhood. For example, in the Tecumseh Study, people in their 40s with elevated blood pressure, as a group, had higher blood pressure readings than normal at the age of 7 years (*23, 35*). While tracking is effective in predicting group experience, the ability to predict adult levels of blood pressure in childhood is limited.

3.4.2 *Genetic factors*

The genetic basis of high blood pressure has been well supported by experimental research, and while some monogenic hypertensive disorders in humans have been described, hypertension for the most part is currently regarded to be polygenic. A large number of candidate genes are being studied, especially the angiotensin II converting enzyme (ACE II) and angiotensinogen gene polymorphisms. The use of molecular genetics may, in the near future, enhance our ability to pay more specific attention to some susceptible individuals.

Several phenotypic characteristics have been investigated in both normotensive and hypertensive individuals, with or without a family history of elevated blood pressure. They include several cation membrane-transport systems (like sodium–potassium co-transport and lithium–potassium co-transport), as well as blood pressure response to salt load, exercise, exposure to cold, mental stress and plasma or urinary levels of various hormones like catecholamines and renin. While several of these have shown a positive relationship with a family history of high blood pressure, they cannot be classified as causal factors (36).

3.4.3 *Early life*

It has been recently suggested that an adverse environment during critical periods of development in fetal life and infancy predisposes an individual to risk factors for cardiovascular disease, including high blood pressure. An inverse relationship between blood pressure and birth weight has been demonstrated in longitudinal studies of children as well as adults (37). While these observations raise interesting possibilities of "fetal programming", evidence of migration studies where patterns of blood pressure appear to be strongly influenced by the environment of the host country indicate that such programming is not the only factor influencing adult blood pressures.

3.4.4 *Other predictors in children*

Apart from tracking, the prediction of future hypertension is being sought by studying the response of blood pressure in children to exercise and weight gain, and the relationship between blood pressure and left ventricular mass as determined by echocardiography.

3.4.5 *Body weight*

Evidence for a direct, strong and consistent relationship between weight and blood pressure emerges from cross-sectional and prospective observational studies. In most studies, being overweight is associated with a twofold to sixfold increase in the risk of developing hypertension (38). The proportion of hypertension attributable to obesity has been estimated to be 30-65% in Western populations. From observational data, multivariate regressions of blood pressure show a rise of 2-3 mmHg (0.13-0.27 kPa) SBP and 1-3 mmHg (0.13-0.4 kPa) DBP for each 10 kg increase in weight.

3.4.6 *Central obesity and the metabolic syndrome*

"Central obesity", indicated by an increased waist to hip ratio, has been positively correlated with high blood pressure in several populations. The co-existence of central obesity, insulin resistance, hyperinsulinaemia, glucose intolerance, dyslipidaemia and hypertension has also been highlighted in recent years (*39-40*). Several studies have noted the association of increased insulin levels with high blood pressure, in both obese and non-obese populations. Furthermore, insulin resistance has been found in otherwise healthy offspring of patients with hypertension and in young, lean, salt-sensitive normotensive subjects, indicating that insulin resistance is present before the development of hypertension in genetically predisposed individuals (*41*).

3.4.7 *Nutritional factors*

Sodium chloride
Experimental as well as observational studies have shown that the intake of sodium chloride, in excess of physiological requirements, is associated with high blood pressure. The strength of the association between urinary sodium excretion and blood pressure increases with age. An overview of 14 population-based studies yielded a pooled regression-slope for SBP and DBP respectively of 3.7 mmHg (0.49 kPa) and 2.0 mmHg (0.27 kPa) per 100 mmol of urinary sodium excretion per day (*42*). In another analysis of 24 observational studies, the calculated slopes for the regression of SBP and DBP respectively on estimated daily sodium intake ranged from 4.9 mmHg (0.65 kPa) and 1.8 mmHg (0.24 kPa) per 100 mmol of sodium in 20-29 year olds to 10.3 mmHg (0.4 kPa) and 2.9 mmHg (0.39 kPa) per 100 mmol of sodium in those aged 60-69 years (*43*).

On the basis of the results of INTERSALT, an interpopulation study involving 10 079 men and women in 52 centres from 32 countries, it has been projected that a 100 mmol/day lower intake of sodium over a lifetime would result in a 9 mmHg (1.2 kPa) smaller rise in systolic pressure from 25 to 55 years of age (*44*). This could correspond by age 55 to a 16% reduction in mortality for coronary heart disease, 23% for stroke and 13% for deaths from all causes (*44*).

Potassium
INTERSALT, CARDIAC and other studies have identified an inverse relationship between blood pressure and dietary intake of potassium (*45, 46*). The INTERSALT study noted a decrease of 2.7 mmHg (0.36 kPa) in SBP for a 60 mmol/day increase in the excretion of urinary potassium. Blood pressure has been more closely related to the ratio of urinary sodium to potassium than to either electrolyte alone. The INTERSALT analysis showed that a reduction of the 24-hour urinary sodium-potassium ratio of 3:1 (170 mmol of sodium/55 mmol of potassium) to

1:1 (70 mmol of sodium/70 mmol of potassium) is associated with a 3.4 mmHg (0.45 kPa) reduction in SBP (*44*).

Other micronutrients
The role of other micronutrients such as calcium, magnesium and zinc in determining blood pressure has been investigated in several population surveys as well as in intervention studies. However, a major independent role for these micronutrients determining the risk of future hypertension has not been established.

Macronutrients
Although observational studies suggest the association of several macronutrients (fat, fatty acids, carbohydrate, fibre and protein) with blood pressure, there is as yet no evidence of a causal relationship with hypertension. There is also little evidence that relatively short-term variations in the intake of macronutrients affect blood pressure in normotensive or mildly hypertensive individuals.

3.4.8 *Alcohol*

Alcohol consumption has been consistently related to high blood pressure in cross-sectional as well as prospective observational studies in several populations. Both acute and chronic effects have been noted and are independent of obesity, smoking, physical activity, sex and age (*47*). While it is not clear whether a threshold effect exists, when two or more drinks are consumed per day SBP rises approximately 1.0 mmHg (0.13 kPa) and DBP approximately 0.5 mmHg (0.07 kPa) per alcoholic drink. Daily drinkers were observed to have SBP and DBP levels respectively of 6.6 mmHg (0.89 kPa) and 4.7 mmHg (0.63 kPa) higher than once-a-week drinkers, independent of the total weekly quantity (*44*).

3.4.9 *Physical activity*

Sedentary and unfit normotensive individuals have a 20–50% increased risk of developing hypertension during follow up when compared with their more active and fit peers (*48*). Regular aerobic physical activity, adequate to achieve at least a moderate level of physical fitness, has been shown to be beneficial for both prevention and treatment of hypertension. The inverse relationship between blood pressure and aerobic physical activity in leisure time persists after adjustment for age, sex, body-mass index and workplace activity.

3.4.10 *Heart rate*

When groups of normotensive and untreated hypertensive subjects, matched for age and sex, are compared, the heart rate of the hypertensive group is invariably higher. This may reflect a resetting of sympathetic activity at a higher level. The role of heart variability in blood pressure needs further research to elucidate whether the relation is causal or prognostic.

3.4.11 *Psychosocial factors*

There is evidence that various forms of acute mental stress increase blood pressure. There is, however, little evidence that long-term stress has long-term effects, independent of confounding factors such as dietary habits and socioeconomic factors. Overall, the available evidence is insufficient to allow definite conclusions of causality or permit quantification of the relative independent risk. Methodologically sound research is needed in this area.

3.4.12 *Environmental factors*

Exposure to noise pollution, air pollution and soft water have all been implicated as risk factors for high blood pressure. Although more research is needed on this, protecting the public from pollution should be a priority on the grounds that it affects health in many other ways besides contributing to hypertension.

4. Pathophysiology of essential hypertension

As summarized in section 3.4, development of hypertension depends on the interaction between genetic predisposition and environmental factors. How this interaction occurs is still incompletely understood. It is known, however, that hypertension is accompanied by functional alterations of the sympathetic (adrenergic) nervous system, the kidney, the renin-angiotensin system and other humoral mechanisms. Hypertension then results in various structural changes of the cardiovascular system that both amplify the hypertensive stimuli and initiate cardiovascular damage. Recent research has called attention to the possible role of endothelial dysfunction in hypertension.

4.1 Sympathetic nervous system

The sympathetic nervous system may play a major role in initiating essential hypertension and may contribute to hypertension related to hyperdynamic circulatory states. Measurements of the concentration of catecholamines in the plasma have been employed to assess sympathetic nervous activity. Several authors have reported increased concentrations of norepinephrine in the plasma of patients with essential hypertension, particularly in younger patients; this has been confirmed by more precise measurements of norepinephrine spillover into the bloodstream (*49*). Recent confirmation comes from studies on sympathetic activity recorded directly from sympathetic nerves of superficial muscle in patients with essential hypertension (*50, 51*). It has also been shown that pressor and depressor reflex responses to baroreceptor manipulation are reset in experimental and clinical forms of hypertension (*52*).

4.2 Renal mechanisms

Renal mechanisms have often been implicated in the pathogenesis of hypertension, either through an altered pressure natriuresis leading to sodium retention or through an altered release of pressor factors (such as renin) or of depressor factors (such as prostaglandins and medullipin) (*53*).

4.3 Renin–angiotensin system

The renin-angiotensin system has a major role in the physiological control of blood pressure and sodium balance. It has important implications in the development of renal hypertension and may be involved in the pathogenesis of essential hypertension. The role of the renin-angiotensin system at the cardiac, vascular and renal level is mediated by the production or activation of several growth factors and vasoactive substances, inducing further vasoconstriction and stimulating cellular hypertrophy (*54*).

4.4 Structural cardiovascular adaptation

The increased load on the vascular system caused by high blood pressure and activation of growth factors leads to structural adaptation with narrowing of the arteriolar lumen and an increase in the media–wall ratio. This amplifies resistance to blood flow and increases vascular responsiveness to vasoconstrictor stimuli (*55*). Vascular adaptation is quite rapid in onset.

Cardiac structural adaptations consist of thickening of the left ventricular wall in response to an increased afterload (concentric hypertrophy), and an increase in left ventricular diameter and a corresponding increase in wall thickness (eccentric hypertrophy) in response to a sustained increase of preload (*56*).

Both vascular and cardiac structural adaptations act as amplifiers of the haemodynamic pattern of hypertension and as initiators of several of the complications of hypertension (*57*).

4.5 Hypertension and endothelial dysfunction

New studies have shown endothelium involvement in the conversion of angiotensin I to angiotensin II, in kinin inactivation and in the production of endothelium-derived relaxing factor or nitric oxide. Furthermore, the endothelium plays a role in the local hormonal and neurogenic control of vascular tone and the haemostatic processes. It also releases vasoconstrictive agents, including endothelin, that may be implicated in some of the vascular complications of hypertension (*58*).

In the presence of hypertension and/or atherosclerosis, endothelial function is often impaired and pressor responses to local or endogenous stimuli may become dominant. It is too early to determine if hypertension in general is associated with significant dysfunction of the endothelium. It is also not yet clear whether endothelial dysfunction is secondary to hypertension, or whether it sometimes precedes it as a primary expression of genetic predisposition.

Recent research has identified more clearly some of the patho-physiological mechanisms involved in hypertension. However, it is still not certain which factors initiate essential hypertension and which perpetuate it. Hypertension appears today to be a more complex condition than it was 20 years ago. A better understanding of the pathophysiological disturbances underlying hypertension and its complications is needed to improve the understanding of what can be achieved by treatment with available antihypertensive agents.

5. Hypertension with identifiable cause

The etiology is unknown in over 95% of cases of elevated blood pressure. In a community study by Liu et al., using the minimum necessary laboratory tests, the cause of hypertension could be identified in only 1.1% of cases (59). Only in hypertensive patients referred to hospital will there be a higher percentage with an identifiable cause (secondary hypertension).

The possible causes of hypertension are classified in Table 4 (60). When considering the incidence of secondary hypertension in the population at large, more attention should be paid to the effects of administering exogenous substances or drugs.

5.1 Hypertension caused by drugs or exogenous substances

Drugs and substances capable of inducing a rise in blood pressure are listed in Table 4. The problem of hormonal contraceptives is discussed in section 7.2.2.

5.2 Hypertension caused by organic disease

5.2.1 Coarctation of the aorta and aortitis

Coarctation of the aorta is a congenital narrowing of the aorta, usually adjacent to the insertion of the ductus arteriosus. It gives rise to a characteristic form of hypertension in which the femoral pulses are diminished or absent and delayed in comparison with the radial pulses. It should be treated by surgical correction of the lesion.

Aortitis is often seen in adolescent girls or young adults in east Asian countries. It presents clinically as moderate to severe hypertension.

Table 4
Classification of hypertension by etiology

A. Essential or primary hypertension

B. Secondary hypertension

1. Induced by exogenous substances or drugs

 Hormonal contraceptives
 Corticosteroids
 Liquorice and carbenoxolone
 Sympathomimetics
 Cocaine
 Tyramine-containing foods and monoamine-oxidase inhibitors
 Non-steroidal anti-inflammatory drugs
 Ciclosporin
 Erythropoietin

2. Associated with renal disorders

 Renal parenchymal disease
  Acute glomerulonephritis
  Chronic nephritis
  Chronic pyelonephritis
  Obstructive nephropathy
  Polycystic diseases
  Connective-tissue disease
  Diabetic nephropathy
  Hydronephrosis
  Congenital hypoplastic kidneys
  Trauma
 Renovascular hypertension
 Renin-producing tumours
 Renoprival hypertension
 Primary sodium retention (Liddle syndrome, Gordon syndrome)

3. Associated with endocrine disorders

 Acromegaly
 Hypothyroidism
 Hypercalcaemia
 Hyperthyroidism
 Adrenal
  Cortical
  (i) Cushing syndrome
  (ii) Primary aldosteronism
  (iii) Congenital adrenal hyperplasia
  Medullary: phaeochromocytoma
 Extra-adrenal chromaffin tumours
 Carcinoid tumours

4. Associated with coarctation of the aorta and aortitis

5. Pregnancy-induced

Table 4 (*continued*)

6. Associated with neurological disorders
    Increased intercranial pressure
        Brain tumour
        Encephalitis
        Respiratory acidosis
    Sleep apnoea
    Quadriplegia
    Acute porphyria
    Familial dysautonomia
    Lead poisoning
    Guillain-Barré syndrome

7. Surgically induced
    Peri-operative hypertension

5.2.2 *Renal disease*

Hypertension is common in patients with renal disease, and may occur even at normal glomerular filtration rate. The major pressor mechanisms are an abnormal pressure–natriuresis relation and inappropriate activity of the renin–angiotensin system.

Bilateral renal disease
Renal parenchymal lesions. In the broad group of diseases caused by these lesions (typically affecting both kidneys), distinct impairment of renal function usually accompanies blood pressure elevation. Examples are: acute or chronic glomerulonephritis; radiation nephritis; nephropathy due to abuse of analgesics (mainly phenacetin); polycystic disease; and chronic pyelonephritis. Drug therapy is necessary to control hypertension, when present, in all these conditions. Chronic glomerulonephritis is the most common cause of secondary hypertension.

Hypertension in patients with advanced renal failure. Studies indicate that intracellular calcium concentrations may be increased early in renal failure, and that this increase occurs in association with both hyperparathyroidism and hypertension. Treatment of hyperparathyroidism with alfacalcidol may result in reductions in both. In patients requiring regular haemodialysis, blood pressure is usually controlled by removal of salt and water during dialysis and by restricting intake between dialysis sessions. In a few instances the addition of antihypertensive drugs is also needed. Occasionally patients develop refractory hypertension despite these measures, with plasma levels of renin and angiotensin II usually becoming very high. Bilateral nephrectomy in these patients permits subsequent control of the blood pressure by dialysis alone.

Hypertension after transplantation. The kidney transplant population has a greater prevalence of correctable forms of hypertension than the general population. Physicians should proceed with a diagnostic assessment of the possible contributions to hypertension of the native kidney, vascular stenosis, chronic rejection, and drug therapy.

Unilateral renal lesions
When such lesions are found in a hypertensive patient, removal of the affected kidney may sometimes reduce the blood pressure. Some of these lesions require excision for reasons other than that of blood pressure control. However, if control of blood pressure is the only reason, careful evaluation is necessary before surgery because a satisfactory reduction does not always result and because the condition may be readily controlled with antihypertensive drugs. Examples of unilateral renal lesions are: hydronephrosis; single cyst; various benign and malignant tumours (including the rare renin-secreting tumour); and unilateral renal tuberculosis.

The initial detection of a unilateral renal lesion is usually made by ultrasound or intravenous pyelography.

Renal artery lesions
The principal lesions causing renal artery stenosis are arteritis in east Asian countries, atheroma and fibromuscular hyperplasia in developed countries. Successful surgical correction of a renal artery stenosis or percutaneous transluminal renal angioplasty may often, though not invariably, alleviate hypertension and thus avoid or reduce the use of antihypertensive agents. Renal artery stenosis may be seen initially as severe and symptomatic hypokalaemia, secondary to excessive aldosterone secretion.

Severe hypertension and renal infarct
Renal infarction, which sometimes follows renal angioplasty, can be complicated by arterial hypertension, which is sometimes severe and may present as hypertensive encephalopathy and epilepsy. Thrombolysis may be helpful in these situations.

Hypertension secondary to renin-secreting juxtaglomerular cell tumour
This is a very rare form of secondary hypertension, characterized by hyper-reninaemia and the presence of a renal mass identifiable by computer-assisted tomography.

5.2.3 Disease of the adrenal cortex

Primary aldosteronism
Primary aldosteronism is a fascinating disease with a logical patho-physiology and a variety of manifestations. It is found in fewer than 0.5% of hypertensive patients.

Primary aldosteronism can be caused by a single adrenocortical adenoma or bilateral adrenocortical hyperplasia, and is associated with an increase in body sodium and a decrease in potassium levels in the plasma. Plasma renin is also suppressed. If the cause is a solitary adenoma, the aldosteronism, and hence the hypertension, may be corrected by surgical excision of the adenoma. Non-adenomatous cases should given long-term treatment with potassium-sparing diuretics; surgical treatment is not recommended.

Glucocorticoid-dependent hypertension
Glucocorticoid excess (Cushing syndrome) is associated with hypertension in at least 70% of patients, independent of the subtype (pituitary or adrenal) and its duration. The mortality of patients with Cushing syndrome is four times that of the general population when matched for age and sex, and much of this excess mortality is caused by cardiovascular disease. Hypertension remits in most of the patients after successful treatment, but may persist in some.

Inborn errors of corticosteroid biosynthesis
Dexamethasone-suppressible hyperaldosteronism is an inherited disease with autosomal-dominant transmission. All its clinical and biochemical abnormalities can be corrected by long-term treatment with dexa-methasone.

New form of mineralocorticoid hypertension. A new form of mineralocorticoid hypertension has been described that arises from impaired metabolism of physiological glucocorticoids, i.e. the in-activation of cortisol to cortisone by the enzyme 11β-hydroxysteroid dehydrogenase. Congenital absence of this enzyme (the syndrome of apparent mineralocorticoid excess) results in cortisol acting as a potent mineralocorticoid. This is also the mechanism by which liquorice and carbenoxolone can raise blood pressure.

5.2.4 Phaeochromocytoma

Overactive adrenal medullary tissue (within or outside the adrenal medulla itself) can produce sustained or paroxysmal hypertension. Phaeochromocytoma is characterized by excessive catecholamine secretion and the definitive treatment is excision of the tumour. In cases of widespread or metastasizing phaeochromocytoma, where surgical excision is not possible, concurrent treatment with both α-adrenoceptor and β-adrenoceptor blocking agents is called for.

Pre-operative localization of the phaeochromocytoma by computer-assisted tomography and by differential determination of plasma levels of catecholamines in the vena cava has proved satisfactory. Mortality from surgery is now less than 3%. Cases of phaeochromocytoma with normal catecholamine levels have also been reported.

5.3 Hypertensive disease of pregnancy

This is covered later in the report in section 7.2.2 on hypertension in women.

5.4 Peri-operative hypertension

The reported prevalence of peri-operative hypertension associated with coronary-artery bypass ranges from 30% to 80%. This wide range may reflect different definitions of hypertension. The consequences of episodes of peri-operative hypertension include bleeding from vascular suture lines, cerebrovascular haemorrhage or subendocardial ischaemia, and are associated with a mortality rate that may approach 50%. Increases in peripheral vascular resistance, caused by elevated levels of circulating catecholamines, appear to be the main mechanism. Prompt antihypertensive therapy is indicated.

6. Organ damage associated with hypertension

Untreated hypertension increases the risk of vascular damage involving both small (resistance) arteries and arterioles and large (conduit) arteries. These lesions lead to cardiac, renal and cerebrovascular morbidity and mortality. The incidence of these different lesions is also dependent upon the level of other risk factors (such as plasma cholesterol, diabetes and tobacco smoking) in the community. In populations of industrialized countries, in which blood lipids are frequently high, most of the morbidity and mortality from hypertension occur from atherosclerotic or cardiac complications. In other areas of the world, like China, the Russian Federation and South America, cerebrovascular accidents are still the most frequent morbid manifestations of hypertension, and malignant or accelerated hypertension is frequently observed. While in the United States of America and in most European countries there has been a continuous decline in mortality by stroke and coronary disease during the past three decades, the incidence of cardiovascular disease is steadily increasing in many developing countries in which programmes for detection, treatment and prevention of hypertension and other risk factors are not implemented.

6.1 Heart

Cardiac complications of hypertension are often grouped together and defined as "hypertensive heart disease". However, these complications are numerous, are related to high blood pressure in different ways, and may be influenced differently by antihypertensive agents. It is preferable not to use a vague, comprehensive term, but rather to refer to each of these complications separately (61).

6.1.1 *Left ventricular hypertrophy*

Left ventricular hypertrophy has long been considered a complication of hypertension. First evaluated anatomically, then radiologically, its electrocardiographic pattern has been established as an independent risk factor, or at least as a marker of additional risk in hypertensive patients (*62*). The risk is considerably greater for the so-called "strain" pattern (changes in the S–T segment and T wave) than for the "voltage" pattern (high-voltage R and S waves) alone and, on the whole, left ventricular hypertrophy is a more powerful predictor of subsequent adverse cardiovascular events than other traditional risk factors (*62*).

The echocardiogram provides a specific and sensitive assessment of left ventricular hypertrophy: left ventricular mass (often normalized to the surface area of the body) can be calculated from the thickness of the septum and posterior wall and the diameter of the left ventricle at the end of diastole; other geometric alterations of the heart can also be measured. Although clinical follow up of patients with left ventricular hypertrophy shown by the echocardiogram (*63, 64*) is rather short, data indicate that the risk of cardiovascular events increases progressively with the degree of hypertrophy. It is not yet known whether this risk is associated with increased myocardial mass, an associated increase in collagen myocardial content (fibrosis) or associated alterations in the coronary circulation (see below). Treatment for hypertension can reverse ventricular hypertrophy, with no impairment of systolic function and improved diastolic function. Whether the additional risk associated with left ventricular hypertrophy also regresses with treatment remains to be established (*61*).

6.1.2 *Diastolic function*

Measurement of the diastolic transmitral flow in the left ventricle by Doppler velocimetry has shown that the ratio of the peak-flow velocity during atrial contraction (A wave) to that during the early diastolic rapid-filling phase (E wave) is frequently elevated in hypertensive subjects compared with normotensive subjects, even in the absence of other structural or functional cardiac alterations. There is no evidence yet that isolated alteration of the diastolic function in hypertension has any clinical relevance or that its therapeutic regression is beneficial (*65*).

6.1.3 *Large and small coronary arteries*

Atherosclerotic plaques are frequently found in the epicardial coronary arteries of hypertensive patients, especially in those in whom other risk factors for atherosclerosis are found, i.e. high plasma lipids and smoking. Prevention or correction of coronary atherosclerosis should not be limited to lowering blood pressure: active intervention against these other risk factors is necessary. In cases of mild hypertension, cessation of smoking may be more effective than reduction of blood pressure in preventing and correcting coronary disease.

There is increasing evidence, however, that coronary flow reserve (i.e. the maximum capacity to increase coronary blood flow) is often reduced by 30–40% in hypertensive patients, even in the absence of stenotic lesions of epicardial coronary arteries. Cardiac biopsy has suggested that structural rather than purely functional alterations of small (resistance) coronary arteries may be largely responsible for this limitation of coronary reserve (66).

It is well known that the incidence of myocardial infarction and sudden cardiac death is increased in hypertension. It is not known at present how much of this increased incidence is due to atherosclerotic lesions of large coronary arteries, left ventricular hypertrophy, myocardial fibrosis or disease of the small coronary arteries (61).

6.1.4 *Congestive heart failure*

Although systolic function is often preserved in hypertension, untreated hypertension may lead to congestive heart failure. Indeed, before treatment became feasible or common, congestive heart failure was one of the commonest complications of hypertension. Progressive dilation of the left ventricle associated with coronary atherosclerosis or disease of the small coronary arteries marks the development of cardiac failure. Meta-analysis of controlled clinical trials, including those on hypertension in the elderly, indicates that antihypertensive therapy can reduce the incidence of congestive heart failure by about 50% (67).

Development of congestive heart failure in hypertensive patients is also dependent on other risk factors; prevention and correction of these additional risk factors will help prevent congestive heart failure. Black hypertensive patients are reported to be especially prone to congestive heart failure, although the reasons for this are not sufficiently understood. In Africa a form of dilated cardiomyopathy with biventricular failure has been described in hypertensive patients. Occasionally, left ventricular failure can be observed in hypertensive patients with small hearts and severe diastolic dysfunction.

6.2 Brain, retina and carotid arteries

6.2.1 *Cerebrovascular disease*

The relation between the incidence of stroke and blood pressure is continuous and particularly steep. All types of stroke (haemorrhagic, lacunar and thrombotic) are associated with hypertension. Antihypertensive treatment has been shown to be particularly effective in reducing the incidence of stroke, a 5-6 mmHg (0.67–0.8 kPa) reduction in diastolic blood pressure reducing incidence by about 40% (9). Plasma cholesterol is not related to the risk of stroke as strongly as hypertension, but tobacco smoking, diabetes and obesity are predictors. Transient ischaemic attacks are also related to hypertension and, in turn, are an important risk factor for a complete stroke. It is not known to what extent these attacks can be prevented by antihypertensive treatment, but intervention trials have shown that the risk of a complete stroke following a transient ischaemic attack can be reduced by antithrombotic therapy.

Vascular dementia is also a common sequela to hypertension in populations of many countries, even where other cardiovascular risk factors (e.g. high levels of blood lipids) seem to be less common.

Despite considerable technical improvements in evaluating cerebrovascular disease (imaging using computer-assisted tomography, nuclear magnetic resonance, radionuclide methods, transcranial Doppler ultrasound, etc.), several problems concerning brain damage and hypertension remain unsolved:

- Are all types of stroke equally prevented by antihypertensive therapy and, in particular, do haemorrhagic and lacunar lesions respond better than infarcts?
- What is the clinical significance of lesions of cerebral white matter in hypertension?
- Can treatment of hypertension significantly reduce the development of vascular dementia?
- Is antihypertensive therapy as valuable in preventing the recurrence of stroke as in primary prevention?
- Is there a therapeutic "window" in the early phase of ischaemic stroke (61)?

6.2.2 *Retina*

Examination of the eye grounds has been a traditional way of evaluating organ damage in hypertensive patients. The classification of Keith, Wagener and Barker has been widely used, but in the past three decades less importance has been placed on minor vascular changes, such as those defined as grades I and II, on the basis that simple thickening of retinal arteries is related more closely to age than to blood pressure (61).

6.2.3 *Carotid arteries*

The well-known increased prevalence of atherosclerotic complications in hypertensive patients is associated with an increased incidence of atherosclerotic lesions in the carotid arteries, especially at the bifurcation. Severe carotid stenoses are known to be a frequent cause of stroke, and ulcerated plaques can be the source of emboli provoking ischaemic strokes or transient ischaemic attacks. The morphology of the carotid arteries, the presence of plaques and their nature and rate of growth, and the extent of stenoses can now be evaluated by non-invasive techniques (echography and Doppler ultrasound) that have largely replaced invasive angiographic techniques (61).

6.3 The kidney

The kidney is an important target of hypertension-induced organ damage. Severe and malignant (accelerated) hypertension often leads to renal insufficiency within a few years, mostly as a consequence of fibrinoid necrosis of small renal arteries. In less severe forms of hypertension, like those prevalent today, renal damage caused by arteriosclerosis is rather mild and develops more slowly (*68*). The development of renal damage in hypertension is commonly heralded by proteinuria. The current definition of proteinuria is a urinary protein excretion of greater than 300 mg a day; the term micro-albuminuria has been coined during the past decade to define an abnormally elevated urinary albumin excretion (30–300 mg/day) in the absence of clinical proteinuria as measured by standard laboratory methods. Proteinuria has been found to be an independent risk factor for mortality from all causes and cardiovascular disease (*69*). Reduction of proteinuria can be achieved by effective blood pressure reduction (*70*). Although antihypertensive treatment can improve renal function in severely hypertensive patients with accelerated renal deterioration, more recent trials of treatment of patients with mild and moderate hypertension have demonstrated little benefit for renal function despite the well-known reduction in the incidence of stroke. This may be because in mild hypertension renal disease progresses too slowly to be significantly appreciated during the relatively short duration of a controlled trial. None the less, hypertension remains a leading cause of renal disease accounting for 15–20% of all cases of renal failure in the United States of America and for 33% in black Americans (*71*).

6.4 Aortic and peripheral artery disease

Hypertension is also associated with aortic atherosclerosis, especially of the abdominal aorta which can lead to aortic aneurysm. A dissecting aneurysm calls for immediate lowering of blood pressure and surgical intervention. Peripheral arterial disease of iliac, femoral and popliteal arteries can also occur in hypertensive patients, particularly those who smoke. Stopping smoking is of paramount importance to avoid or correct peripheral vascular disease.

7. Clinical assessment of the hypertensive patient

7.1 Diagnostic procedures

7.1.1 *Goals and methods*

The diagnostic investigation of a subject in whom high blood pressure has been found has several goals:

- confirm a chronic elevation of blood pressure
- assess the overall cardiovascular risk
- evaluate existing organ damage or concomitant disease
- search for possible causes.

Obviously, all these distinct goals are elements of a single, coherent, step-wise diagnostic process using the three classic methods: history-taking, physical examination and laboratory investigation. The extent of laboratory investigation can be adjusted according to the evidence obtained by history, physical examination and preliminary laboratory tests.

The principal difficulty during the diagnostic process is to determine the extent of investigation. A superficial investigation is unacceptable since hypertension is a life-long disease and therapy may have serious implications for the patient. On the other hand, the patient should not be exposed to a series of unjustified examinations. Sound judgement has to be applied (*12, 72*).

7.1.2 *Blood pressure measurement*

Blood pressure is commonly measured by a physician or nurse in an outpatient clinic by a mercury manometer using the auscultatory method. Before confirming the presence of hypertension and grading it as mild (grade 1), moderate (grade 2) or severe (grade 3), elevated blood pressure levels must be confirmed several times. The interval for rechecking is determined by the initial blood pressure measurement. Table 5 gives recommendations for follow-up measurements. Blood pressure measurement is covered in full in section 2.2.

The scheduling of follow up should be modified by reliable information about past blood pressure measurements, other cardiovascular risk factors, and target-organ damage.

Table 5
Recommended follow up based on initial screening blood pressure[a]

Blood pressure, mmHg (kPa)		
Systolic	Diastolic	Recommended follow up
<130 (17.3)	<85 (11.3)	Recheck in 2 years
130–140 (17.3–18.7)	85–90 (11.3–12.0)	Recheck in 1 year
140–180 (18.7–24.0)	90–105 (12.0–14.0)	Mild hypertension (grade 1): confirm repeatedly over a period of at least 3 months
180–210 (24.0–28.0)	105–120 (14.0–16.0)	Moderate hypertension (grade 2): confirm and evaluate promptly and initiate treatment within a few weeks
>210 (28.0)	>120 (16.0)	Severe hypertension (grade 3): evaluate and treat immediately

[a] If the systolic and diastolic categories are different, follow recommendations for the shortest follow-up interval.

Blood pressure assessment can also be supported by blood pressure measurements taken at home, provided the differences between clinic and home readings are considered (see section 2.2.3). Monitoring ambulatory blood pressure can be useful in a few specific cases, particularly when:

- there is an unusually large discrepancy between blood pressure values measured in the clinic and at home;
- there is a marked discrepancy between the elevation of blood pressure values and the absence of signs of organ damage;
- there are marked differences between clinic blood pressure values measured on different occasions;
- there is resistance to treatment.

In all these cases, attention should be paid to the evidence that average values for ambulatory blood pressure measured over 24 hours are commonly several mmHg lower than clinic blood pressure, especially in the elderly.

7.1.3 *History-taking*

Careful taking of a patient's history helps in providing important information about concomitant risk factors, symptoms of organ damage and hints of secondary hypertension. Table 6 indicates the type of information that should be sought.

7.1.4 *Physical examination*

Accurate physical examination should concentrate on finding possible signs of organ damage and signs suggesting secondary hypertension, as indicated in Table 7.

7.1.5 *Laboratory investigation*

A detailed history and physical examination help to indicate the laboratory investigations needed; these tests will be relatively simple in the majority of patients with mild or moderate hypertension and more detailed in those with severe or complicated hypertension. Full laboratory investigation may not be necessary or useful in certain patients. It may entail unnecessary discomfort and risk, and may be excessively costly for the community or individual. Detailed evaluation with complex investigations should be reserved for patients with severe or resistant hypertension.

The minimum laboratory investigation needed is a matter of debate. However, it is agreed that investigations should progress from the most simple to the more complicated. It is always better to repeat simple tests for which the results are doubtful, rather than to perform a complex investigation at an early stage. The younger the patient, the higher the blood pressure and the faster the development of hypertension, the more

Table 6
Guidelines for patient history

Risk factors

Family history of hypertension and cardiovascular disease

Family and personal history of hyperlipidaemia

Family and personal history of diabetes mellitus

Smoking habits

Dietary habits

Obesity; amount of physical exercise

Personality of the patient; social environment

Indications of secondary hypertension

Family history of renal disease (polycystic kidney)

Renal disease, urinary tract infection, haematuria, analgesic abuse (parenchymal renal disease)

Drug/substance intake: oral contraceptives, liquorice, carbenoxolone, nasal drops, cocaine, non-steroidal anti-inflammatory drugs, etc.

Episodes of sweating, headache, anxiety (phaeochromocytoma)

Episodes of muscle weakness and tetany (aldosteronism)

Symptoms of organ damage

Brain and eyes: headache, vertigo, impaired vision, transient ischaemic attacks, sensory or motor deficit

Heart: palpitations, chest pain, shortness of breath, swollen ankles

Kidney: thirst, polyuria, nocturia, haematuria

Peripheral arteries: cold extremities, intermittent claudication

detailed the diagnostic examination should be – and the more assiduous the search for potentially curable causes of arterial hypertension.

Laboratory investigations are classified as follows and described in detail in the subsequent pages:

- *Strongly recommended tests:* to be performed on all hypertensive patients. These tests are simple and cheap yet provide basic information about additional risk factors and renal and cardiac function.
- *Additional tests:* other simple tests that may be usefully performed when the facilities are available and additional information is desirable.

Table 7
Physical examination for secondary hypertension and organ damage

Signs suggesting secondary hypertension

Features of Cushing syndrome

Skin stigmata of neurofibromatosis (phaeochromocytoma)

Palpation of enlarged kidneys (polycystic kidney)

Auscultation of abdominal murmurs (renovascular hypertension)

Auscultation of precordial or chest murmurs (aortic coarctation or aortitis)

Diminished and delayed femoral pulses and reduced femoral blood pressure (aortic coarctation or aortitis)

Signs of organ damage

Brain: murmurs over neck arteries, motor or sensory defects

Retina: fundoscopic abnormalities

Heart: location and characteristics of apical impulse, abnormal cardiac rhythms, ventricular gallop, pulmonary rales, dependent oedema

Peripheral arteries: absence, reduction, or asymmetry of pulses, cold extremities, ischaemic skin lesions

---

- *Extended evaluation:* performed by the hospital physician or specialist for a more detailed study of complicated hypertension or to search for a curable cause of hypertension whenever the history, physical examination or simpler tests suggest this possibility.

A list of laboratory investigations is presented in Table 8.

7.2   Hypertension in special populations

7.2.1 *Children and adolescents*

There is no prospective therapeutic study of hypertensive children and adolescents. Reliance must therefore be placed on an epidemiological definition. According to the *Report of the Second Task Force on Blood Pressure Control in Children (73)*, hypertension in the young is defined as average systolic and/or diastolic blood pressure equal to or greater than the 95th percentile for age on at least three occasions. The values are indicated in Table 9.

In a number of adolescents and young people isolated systolic hypertension can be found that has a different causal mechanism than in elderly people (hyperdynamic circulation rather than decreased arterial compliance).

Table 8
Laboratory investigations

Strongly recommended tests

Urine analysis (dipstick test complemented by urinary sediment examination)

Plasma creatinine

Plasma potassium (sodium is often measured in the same sample)

Blood glucose

Serum cholesterol

Electrocardiogram

Additional tests

Fasting plasma triglycerides and high-density lipoprotein-cholesterol

Plasma uric acid

Haemoglobin and haematocrit

Urine culture

Chest X-ray

Echocardiogram

Extended evaluation (domain of the specialist)

Complicated hypertension: tests of cerebral, cardiac and renal function

Search for secondary hypertension: measurement of renin, angiotensin, aldosterone, corticosteroids, catecholamines; aortography and renal arteriography; renal and adrenal ultrasound; computer-assisted tomography (CAT); etc.

Children, like adults, require repeated measurements with proper equipment to determine blood pressure accurately. The widest cuff that will comfortably encircle the arm without covering the cubital fossa should be used. The Korotkoff phase IV sound gives the best indication of diastolic pressure in children because the arterial sound may persist until the cuff pressure has fallen to zero. For infants in whom the accuracy of the measurements by auscultation is uncertain, an electronic device using the Doppler technique can be used. It is important to obtain the confidence of a child before taking a measurement and to ensure that the surroundings are quiet. The prevalence of hypertension is at least 1% in children and increases in adolescents. Physicians who care for children and adolescents are encouraged to measure blood pressure, especially when there is a family history of hypertension, as family clustering is well known.

The higher the blood pressure and the younger the child, the greater the possibility of secondary hypertension. In such cases, risk factors for

Table 9
Classification of hypertension in children and adolescents by age group[a]

Age	Systolic and diastolic blood pressure (SBP and DBP), mmHg (kPa)		
	High to normal[b]	Significant hypertension[c]	Severe hypertension[d]
7 days		SBP 96-105 (12.8-14.0)	SBP≥106 (14.1)
8-30 days		SBP 104-109 (13.9-14.5)	SBP≥110 (14.7)
≤2 years	SBP 104-111 (14.0-14.8)	SBP 112-117 (14.9-15.6)	SBP≥118 (15.7)
	DBP 70-73 (9.33-9.73)	DBP 74-81 (9.86-10.8)	DBP≥82 (10.9)
3-5 years	SBP 108-115 (14.4-15.3)	SBP 116-123 (15.5-16.4)	SBP≥124 (16.5)
	DBP 70-75 (9.33-10.0)	DBP 76-83 (10.1-11.1)	DBP≥84 (11.2)
6-9 years	SBP 114-121 (15.2-16.1)	SBP 122-129 (16.3-17.2)	SBP≥130 (17.3)
	DBP 74-77 (9.86-10.3)	DBP 78-85 (10.4-11.3)	DBP≥86 (11.5)
10-12 years	SBP 122-125 (16.3-16.6)	SBP 126-133 (16.8-17.7)	SBP≥134 (17.9)
	DBP 78-81 (10.4-10.8)	DBP 82-89 (10.9-11.9)	DBP≥90 (12.0)
13-15 years	SBP 130-135 (17.3-18.0)	SBP 136-143 (18.1-19.05)	SBP≥144 (19.2)
	DBP 80-85 (10.7-11.3)	DBP 86-91 (11.5-12.1)	DBP≥92 (12.3)
16-18 years	SBP 136-141 (18.1-18.8)	SBP 142-149 (18.9-19.8)	SBP≥150 (20.0)
	DBP 84-91 (11.2-12.1)	DBP 92-97 (12.3-12.9)	DBP≥98 (13.1)

[a] Adapted from Task Force on Blood Pressure Control in Children (73); by permission of *Pediatrics*, 79:1-25, copyright 1987. Note that adult classifications differ.
[b] 90-94th percentile.
[c] 95-99th percentile.
[d] >99th percentile.

secondary hypertension should be assessed, including family history, obesity, diet and level of physical activity. In adolescents, use of alcohol, cocaine or other addictive substances should be considered as a possible cause of elevated blood pressure. Laboratory tests for young patients are generally similar to those recommended for adults. However, efforts to arrive at a diagnosis of secondary hypertension should be more thorough in a child.

The underlying cause, severity or complications of hypertension in children will determine the degree and types of intervention required. Therapy should reduce blood pressure without causing adverse effects that limit compliance or impair normal growth and development. Initial treatment should consist of lifestyle modifications but this may be insufficient when hypertension is severe or when there is a demonstrable cause not associated with lifestyle.

Weight reduction in obese children often reduces blood pressure. Antihypertensive drug therapy should usually be reserved for children with blood pressure above the 99th percentile or with significantly elevated blood pressure that responds inadequately to lifestyle modifications or is associated with target-organ damage. Pharmacological agents generally used for adults are also effective in young people. There is no evidence that isolated mild systolic hypertension in adolescents and young people should be treated, other than with lifestyle counselling. Uncomplicated elevated blood pressure, by itself, should not be a reason to restrict asymptomatic children and adolescents from participating in physical activities, particularly because isotonic (phasic) exercise may both prevent and relieve hypertension.

7.2.2 *Women*

Sex differences in the control of blood pressure and outcomes
Long-term and large clinical trials of antihypertensive treatment have included both men and women but have not clearly demonstrated sex differences in blood pressure response and outcomes. Because the rate of cardiovascular events in middle-aged women is much lower than in men, these trials had limited power to distinguish the degree of benefit from treatments in men and women. Besides, these trials were not specifically designed to answer the question of treatment efficacy for women. Thus, the failure to demonstrate unequivocally that benefit does exist by retrospective subgroup analysis cannot be taken to mean that drug therapy is not of benefit. Recent trials in older people (*10, 11*) support a similar approach to the management of hypertension in men and women. Further study is needed in this area.

Hypertension associated with oral contraceptives
Prospective controlled studies have shown that estrogen–progestogen oral contraceptives (containing 50 μg or more of estrogen) cause a distinct increase in systolic, and to a lesser extent diastolic, pressure in virtually all women (*74*). In some women marked elevation of blood pressure can occasionally occur. The mechanism of the rise in blood pressure is imperfectly understood. Almost invariably the pressure falls when the oral contraceptive is withdrawn, but this may take six or more months. It is not known whether hormonal contraceptives with lower estrogen content or containing only progestogen cause a similar rise in blood pressure. Alternative methods of contraception should be

considered for hypertensive women, especially as oral contraceptives containing estrogen and progestogen also carry other cardiovascular risks.

Hormone replacement therapy is being increasingly used to prevent osteoporosis in post-menopausal women. There is evidence that replacement with estrogen alone reduces coronary risk (75), but less evidence for this with combined estrogen–progestogen therapy. Such combinations are generally recommended for women with an intact uterus to protect against uterine malignancy. The use of hormone replacement therapy is not contraindicated for women with hypertension, but blood pressure should be monitored frequently as it is not yet clear whether a hypertensive response may occur in some.

Hypertension in pregnancy

The hypertensive disease of pregnancy (76) (variously termed toxaemia of pregnancy, pre-eclampsia, eclampsia and hypertension gestosis) is the major cause of premature birth and perinatal death, and is also responsible for 20–33% of all maternal deaths. It is a major health problem in developing countries. Infants of mothers who have hypertension with proteinuria in late pregnancy are small and are more often stillborn or have a high risk of dying in the neonatal period. The reported incidence of this disease varies widely. Most information derives from hospital studies, which are not representative of the total population. A reasonable estimation is that less than 5% of pregnancies are complicated by clinically relevant blood pressure elevation.

Diagnosis and classification. Hypertension in pregnancy is defined on the basis of DBP measurement by sphygmomanometry using phase IV Korotkoff sounds in women lying on their sides at an angle of 15–30° to the horizontal (the posture of choice) in order to eliminate the haemodynamic changes associated with pregnancy (77); diagnosis of hypertension requires two consecutive measurements of 90 mmHg (12.0 kPa) or more, four or more hours apart, or one measurement of 100 mmHg (13.3 kPa) or more. As DBP values are approximately 10 mmHg (1.33 kPa) lower than non-pregnant values throughout pregnancy, DBP of greater than 85 mmHg (11.3 kPa) should already be considered abnormal.

Classification of the hypertensive disorders of pregnancy into four categories is based upon the clinical findings of hypertension and/or proteinuria during pregnancy:

- pre-eclampsia/eclampsia
- chronic hypertension of whatever cause
- chronic hypertension with superimposed pre-eclampsia/eclampsia
- transient or late hypertension.

Pre-eclampsia/eclampsia. Pre-eclampsia/eclampsia is characterized by hypertension with proteinuria (>300 mg/day) and, at times, coagulation abnormalities or liver abnormalities or both. Oedema is no longer used as a criterion. It occurs primarily in a woman's first pregnancy after the 20th week of gestation and most frequently near to full term. Pre-eclampsia may progress rapidly without warning to the convulsive phase known as eclampsia. Differentiating mild from severe pre-eclampsia may be dangerously misleading, because one quarter of women with eclampsia have "mild" disease or minimal elevations of blood pressure before convulsing.

Prophylactic use of low-dose aspirin is based upon the theory of an imbalance between vasoconstrictor and vasodilator eicosanoid synthesis, but should not be used as a routine until results of several ongoing large, multicentre trials are available.

Women suspected of having eclampsia should be admitted to hospital. If pre-eclampsia or severe hypertension occurs beyond the 36th week of gestation, delivery is the therapy of choice. When problems arise earlier, delivery may be delayed in selected patients under strict supervision. If there is evidence of advanced disease (especially with thrombocytopenia or abnormal liver function tests) or signs or symptoms of impending eclampsia, delivery is indicated regardless of the length of gestation.

For acute, severe hypertension – with DBP of, or greater than, 105 mmHg (14.0 kPa) – in pre-eclampsia/eclampsia, intravenous hydralazine is indicated, aiming for a gradual reduction of DBP to 90-100 mmHg (12.0-13.3 kPa). Magnesium sulfate remains the treatment of choice to prevent eclamptic convulsions.

Chronic hypertension in pregnancy. The diagnosis of chronic hypertension rests on the evidence of raised blood pressure before pregnancy or before the 20th week of gestation. The vast majority of patients in this category have mild to moderate, uncomplicated hypertension, and a benign course of pregnancy. Drug therapy for chronic hypertension in pregnancy remains controversial. If DBP is greater than 95 mmHg (12.7 kPa), methyldopa and β-blockers are the safest agents, although β-blockers may retard fetal growth. Diuretics can be used transiently when blood pressure is difficult to control. Sodium restriction is not recommended. Bed rest may be useful. Inhibitors of angiotensin converting enzyme are contraindicated because of serious fetal and neonatal complications which can be fatal. All inadequately studied antihypertensive drugs are prohibited in pregnancy. For poorly controlled hypertension, the mother's well-being takes precedence over the fetus, and she should be treated as if she were not pregnant if the pharmacological approaches indicated above fail. Pre-eclampsia and eclampsia superimposed on chronic hypertension should be dealt with as mentioned above.

Late or transient hypertension. This condition is characterized by the development of hypertension alone during the later stages of pregnancy, or in the early puerperium, accompanied by a return to normal blood pressure within 10 days of delivery. Long-term follow up of women with a hypertensive pregnancy is important, since a significant proportion will later develop chronic (essential) hypertension.

7.2.3 *Elderly people*

Hypertension is more frequent in people aged 65 years or older, among whom isolated systolic hypertension is particularly frequent. Pseudo-hypertension is sometimes encountered in elderly patients who have such rigid brachial arteries that they cannot be compressed by the sphygmo-manometer cuff, giving falsely high readings. The sudden onset of hypertension in elderly subjects suggests the presence of atherosclerotic renovascular disease.

In absolute terms, hypertension is a much greater risk factor of cardiovascular events in the elderly than in younger people. In developed countries the 10-year risk of a major cardiovascular event ranges from less than 1% in individuals aged 25–34 years to greater than 30% in those aged 65–74 years (*78*). Correspondingly, numerous intervention trials have shown that the absolute benefit of antihypertensive therapy is particularly high in the elderly (*10, 11, 14, 15*).

In addition to the results of the European Working Party on High Blood Pressure in the Elderly (*14*), which clearly demonstrated the beneficial effect of antihypertensive medication, the results of three prospective placebo-controlled therapeutic trials in elderly hypertensive patients all demonstrated a significant reduction of cardiovascular morbidity or mortality (*10, 11, 15*). The SHEP (Systolic Hypertension in the Elderly) Cooperative Research Group (*10*) specifically examined the value of antihypertensive treatment in men and women over 60 years old with iso-lated systolic hypertension, i.e. SBP of 160–219 mmHg (21.3–29.2 kPa) and DBP greater than 90 mmHg (12.0 kPa); highly significant reductions in fatal and non-fatal cardiovascular events were observed, reducing cardiovascular morbidity and mortality to at least the same extent (about 20–50%) as in young and middle-aged patients. Furthermore, since the incidence of cardiovascular events is high in the elderly, the same relative reduction of morbidity and mortality results in a greater absolute benefit in this age group than in younger patients (*12*).

According to the STOP-Hypertension study carried out by Dahlöf et al. (*15*), significant benefits also result from treating the "older elderly" (80 years of age and older). However, in the oldest patients drugs should be used with caution, especially if medication is also prescribed for associated diseases. Efforts should be made to avoid sudden drops in blood pressure and orthostatic hypotension in elderly patients. It should also be remembered that in elderly patients high blood pressure can often be controlled by low-dose medication. Bearing in mind these precautions, the same general guidelines for antihypertensive therapy can be followed for elderly patients as for the young and middle-aged (*72*).

However, treatment of hypertension should be in the context of the overall clinical picture as elderly patients often have other, non-cardiovascular diseases.

7.2.4 *Hypertensive patients with diabetes*

The coexistence of hypertension and non-insulin-dependent diabetes mellitus is common (*79*). Patients with both of these conditions are especially vulnerable to cardiovascular and renal complications; therefore, the control of hypertension and dyslipidaemia – and the cessation of smoking – are particularly important. In patients with incipient diabetic nephropathy, treatment may be instituted at systolic and diastolic blood pressure values as low as 130 mmHg (17.3 kPa) and 85 mmHg (11.3 kPa) respectively.

Lifestyle modifications are beneficial for control of hyperglycaemia, dyslipidaemia and hypertension, which often occur in obese patients with insulin resistance. The syndrome of insulin resistance, characterized by hypertension, dyslipidaemia, hyperinsulinaemia, glucose intolerance and frequently central obesity (*40*), very closely parallels non-insulin-dependent diabetes mellitus. Insulin sensitivity can be improved by weight reduction and exercise. The relation between insulin resistance, glucose intolerance and blood pressure can be traced even in children with normal blood pressure and may be hereditary.

No antihypertensive agent is absolutely contraindicated for use in the diabetic population, but caution is needed with several of them. In particular, diuretics may worsen glucose tolerance; β-blockers may also worsen glucose tolerance, mask the symptoms and prolong recovery from hypoglycaemia.

8. Prevention and control of hypertension in populations

8.1 Rationale

The prevention of complications resulting from high blood pressure in any population requires reducing the risk of developing high blood pressure in the population as a whole (population approach); and identifying individuals with high blood pressure who are at increased risk of developing complications (individual approach). Hypertension in this context is used to denote all levels of elevated blood pressure associated with increased risk of complications and not only those in need of special antihypertensive treatment.

The combination of the individual approach with the population approach, which seeks to control the causes of hypertension (*80*), provides a comprehensive strategy for the prevention and control of hypertension. The two approaches have a synergistic effect: the detection and treatment of individuals heightens community awareness of the problem and facilitates the implementation of a population-based strategy, while changes in population behaviour facilitate adherence to lifestyle interventions by individual patients.

The rationale of the individual approach is clear since both the risks of high blood pressure and the benefits of effective intervention to reduce it have been convincingly demonstrated over a wide range of high blood pressure. The greater the cumulative risk of cardiovascular events and other adverse outcomes, the greater the benefit of effective blood pressure reduction and the greater the need for early and effective intervention.

However, as evident from Fig. 2 (page 13), this approach alone will not prevent all of the cardiovascular–renal disease related to blood pressure in the community. Because there is a continuous relation between blood pressure and cardiovascular disease, complications can occur even within the conventionally defined normotensive range. It is clear from the MRFIT screening cohort follow-up data that even under optimal conditions (which are seldom achieved), the treatment and control of hypertension will influence no more than 70% of the cardiovascular disease related to blood pressure in the community (21).

In the NHANES III survey in the United States of America, 35% of the participants with an SBP of, or greater than, 140 mmHg (18.7 kPa) or a DBP of, or greater than, 90 mmHg (12.0 kPa) reported a lack of awareness of their raised blood pressure; only 49% of those with high blood pressure were receiving drug therapy; and only 21% of those treated had SBP/DBP less than 140/90 mmHg (18.7/12.0 kPa) (23). Similar data are available from other countries. Intervention may also occur late in the natural history of the disease and may not completely eliminate the risk of complications. Thus patients with hypertension who have received treatment still have a higher risk of morbidity and mortality than their untreated "normotensive" counterparts. In addition, the possible adverse effects of drugs may reduce the benefits of treatment and in some countries the costs of therapy may adversely affect compliance.

Thus identification and treatment of clinically hypertensive subjects in a population requires a continued commitment of a high level of health care resources for both the providers and the patients. However, this does not result in a complete reduction of risk and is unsuccessful in altering the risk of future hypertension in large segments of the population. Primary prevention of high blood pressure is therefore also necessary.

From the perspective of developing countries, the prevention of hypertension is imperative. These are societies in epidemiological transition, with deleterious changes in lifestyle accompanying economic development. Major epidemics of cardiovascular disease have been projected to occur, or are already occurring, in these countries.

Campaigns for mass screening, case detection and compliance to long-term drug therapy will face the formidable, if not insurmountable, barriers of prohibitive costs, inadequate or overburdened health infrastructure and socioeconomic constraints that severely curtail the continued commitment of scarce family or governmental resources. Even at present, these countries are grappling with the double burden of persistent pre-transitional problems (infections, malnutrition) and increases in post-transitional disease (cardiovascular disease, cancers), while trying to cope with the threat of AIDS. Hence, the containment of an established epidemic of high blood pressure faces great obstacles in such an environment where health care resources will be scarce and widely dispersed.

The fact that the distribution of blood pressure in many developing countries is to the left of that in developed countries makes the task principally one of preventing a shift to the right. This will probably be easier than achieving a shift to the left in developed countries. This makes primary prevention the major goal in developing countries, using a population-based strategy encouraging changes in lifestyle.

8.2 Prevention of blood pressure elevation

In any population and, therefore, the individual members of that population, the prevention of elevated blood pressure is principally linked to the elimination of modifiable risk factors that contribute to its rise, and promotion of protective factors that help maintain blood pressure in the desirable range associated with low risk of complications.

This approach attempts to shift the whole blood pressure distribution to the left by altering the norms of behaviour within the population. There are large, theoretical advantages to this approach: it attempts to remove the underlying causes of hypertension (and other risks) associated with lifestyle from the population as a whole; it helps individuals to adopt a healthier lifestyle by keeping a normal body weight, eating less salt, consuming less alcohol and increasing physical activity because they will share this behaviour with many other people; and industry, restaurants and shops are encouraged to provide healthier food to meet increased demand.

There are, however, several drawbacks. Since the approach provides only a relatively small preventive benefit to each individual, particularly in the short term, some might be poorly motivated to change behaviour. Furthermore, the physician may also be poorly motivated because the benefit of treatment is rather limited for an individual whose risk is not great.

However, changes in behaviour such as cessation of tobacco smoking and improved diet have been achieved in some communities, producing benefits across the whole spectrum of blood pressure distribution. Since most of the adults in developed countries have blood pressures above the optimal levels, even a small reduction has the potential to produce not only a substantial reduction in prevalence of hypertension but a surprisingly large decrease in cardiovascular risk. It has been estimated that a 2 mmHg (0.27 kPa) downward shift in the entire distribution of SBP is likely to reduce the annual mortality from stroke by 6%, coronary heart disease by 4% and all causes by 3%. The corresponding benefits for a 3 mmHg (0.4 kPa) downward shift in SBP have been estimated to be 8%, 5% and 4% respectively (*44*).

Encouraging changes in behaviour in communities and individuals requires a collaborative effort between health professionals, policy makers, industry, media and other opinion formers as well as a sustained education campaign that targets all sections of the community and all ages.

8.3 Detection and treatment of established hypertension

The individual approach focusing on people at high risk has certain advantages over the population approach: it addresses a problem highly relevant to the individual, and it is associated with high levels of motivation for both the physician and the patient. In addition the use of resources is usually cost-effective.

However, there are also some limitations. Finding the "high-risk" individuals can be difficult and costly. A large number of borderline cases are usually discovered who require a different therapeutic approach to those at high risk. While complications of high blood pressure are reduced in treated hypertensive patients, the individual approach does not influence the incidence of new cases. The costs to society are, therefore, recurring.

8.4 Measures for controlling hypertension

8.4.1 *General measures*

When strategies to control hypertension are being developed, the following issues need to be addressed.

1. In order to formulate priorities and plan public health strategies in individual countries, valid and representative estimates are needed of:
   – the prevalence of high blood pressure
   – other risk factors for cardiovascular disease that contribute to the risk of complications associated with high blood pressure
   – the risk factors leading to the development of high blood pressure.

   Where such data are presently not available, surveys of cardiovascular risk factors should be conducted in population samples.

2. Individuals with high blood pressure should be identified and treated with appropriate interventions early in the natural history of their disease. Although mass screening is neither appropriate nor feasible,

every opportunity for detecting high blood pressure in various health care settings should be used, and self-referral encouraged by increasing public awareness.

3. The health care system must be capable of providing appropriate management to reduce high blood pressure in individuals as well as promoting measures to prevent it in the population.

4. Programmes to control high blood pressure must integrate measures to facilitate appropriate lifestyle changes and provide effective drug therapy when required.

5. The community must be empowered, through education, to contribute effectively to the prevention and control of high blood pressure. This will ensure that control measures are participatory rather than prescriptive.

8.4.2 *Lifestyle measures*

Lifestyle measures for lowering blood pressure
Lifestyle measures are applicable to both the population approach and the individual approach. In the individual patient they are helpful in lowering blood pressure, avoiding or reducing the need for antihypertensive drugs and controlling associated risk factors. In the population, they are of benefit in reducing the risk of developing high blood pressure and other lifestyle-related disorders. However, it is also appreciated that long-term lifestyle changes are difficult to maintain, and it is important that improved knowledge in behavioural modification and maintenance is sought.

Proof of the benefit conferred by lifestyle interventions in lowering blood pressure in hypertensive patients is available from clinical trials evaluating individual risk factors or a combination of risk factors (*81*). Benefits of primary prevention are suggested by ecological studies of trends of risk factors and disease rates in different countries (e.g. the United States of America), demonstration projects (e.g. in North Karelia in Finland) and trials evaluating single-factor and multifactor interventions.

The evidence of associated risk for various environmental factors and the efficacy of interventions aimed at modifying them in treating or preventing high blood pressure have been critically appraised (*13, 23, 47, 82*). Interventions that clearly lower blood pressure are weight reduction, reduced alcohol intake, increased physical activity and reduced sodium intake. Interventions with limited or unproven efficacy include stress management, micronutrient alteration and dietary supplementation with potassium, fish oil, calcium, magnesium or fibre.

Weight reduction. Raised blood pressure is closely correlated with increased body weight. In particular, the accumulation of fat on the trunk or abdomen is closely correlated with hypertension, hyperlipidaemia and diabetes. Weight reduction lowers blood pressure in the majority of hypertensive patients who are more than 10% overweight, and also has beneficial effects on associated risk factors such as the lipid profile and insulin resistance. Overweight hypertensive patients should therefore be counselled to undertake a structured and supervised weight-reduction programme by reducing dietary energy intake and increasing energy expenditure through regular physical exercise. Such a programme should be maintained for 3-6 months in patients with mild or borderline hypertension before antihypertensive drugs are prescribed. Long-term weight reduction, though more difficult to maintain, should be the aim.

Three large controlled trials have demonstrated the effect of weight loss on the primary prevention of hypertension. In the TOHP-1 study of non-pharmacological interventions in people with high to normal blood pressure, mean weight losses in men and women were 4.7 kg and 1.6 kg respectively at 18 months (*81-83*). The corresponding mean SBP/DBP reductions were 3.2/2.8 mmHg (0.43/0.37 kPa) in men and 2.0/1.1 mmHg (0.27/0.15 kPa) in women.

The associations of obesity with abnormalities in serum lipids and insulin and glucose metabolism reinforce the value of the control of obesity as a lifestyle intervention for blood pressure reduction.

Reduction of alcohol intake. Regular alcohol consumption raises blood pressure in both men and women in different ethnic groups, and contributes significantly to the prevalence of hypertension in populations where drinking is a habit. Reduction of alcohol intake over a period of 1-4 weeks results in lowering of blood pressure. Moderating alcohol intake and reducing excess weight have cumulative effects in reducing overall cardiovascular risk.

Randomized cross-over studies showed that reducing alcohol intake by 80-85% resulted in an SBP/DBP reduction of 5.0/3.0 mmHg (0.67/0.4 kPa) in hypertensive subjects and 3.8/1.4 mmHg (0.51/0.19 kPa) in those with normal blood pressure (*84*). A randomized factorial study revealed that restricted alcohol intake alone led to an SBP/DBP reduction of 4.8/3.3 mmHg (0.64/0.44 kPa), while combined alcohol and energy restrictions resulted in an average reduction of 10.2/7.5 mmHg (1.36/1.00 kPa) and a weight loss of 10 kg (*85*).

Increased physical activity. Regular exercise may be beneficial for both prevention and treatment of hypertension. Sedentary and unfit normo-tensive individuals have a 20-50% higher risk of developing hyper-tension than those who are more active (*86*).

Exercise lowers systolic and diastolic blood pressure by 5-10 mmHg (0.67-1.3 kPa) (*87*). Dynamic isotonic exercise such as walking is more effective than static isometric exercise such as weight lifting. Milder levels of exercise, such as brisk walking for 30-60 minutes a day or 3-5 times a week, is possibly better than more strenuous forms of exercise such as running.

Analysis of 22 studies (of which ten included normotensive subjects and seven involved only normotensive subjects) revealed that, in methodologically adequate studies, a mean reduction in SBP of 6.4 mmHg (0.85 kPa) and DBP of 6.9 mmHg (0.92 kPa) was achieved through prescribed exercise (*81*). Another analysis of 30 randomized controlled trials of lower extremity aerobic exercise revealed a 3 mmHg (0.4 kPa) reduction in SBP and DBP (*88*). Thus, the beneficial effects of exercise, though modest, are useful in lowering blood pressure for purposes of prevention as well as control.

Reduced sodium intake. Both epidemiological observations and clinical trials show an association between dietary sodium intake and blood pressure (*45, 89*). Individuals vary substantially in their responses to changes in dietary sodium chloride. Black and elderly people may be more sensitive to salt reduction. An average intake below 6 g of sodium chloride a day should be the aim.

Meta-analysis of 18 clinical trials in hypertensive subjects revealed an SBP/DBP reduction of 4.9/2.6 mmHg (0.65/0.35 kPa) in 1-2 months, associated with a 56-105 mmol reduction in daily sodium intake (*90*). A larger analysis of 78 trials of sodium restriction, one quarter of which included normotensive subjects, demonstrated that observed and predicted blood pressure reductions were most similar in trials lasting over five weeks, suggesting that the effects of sodium restriction may take several weeks to become evident (*91*).

Lifestyle measures for the treatment of associated risk factors
Cessation of tobacco smoking. Although tobacco smoking is not causally related to hypertension, it is a major cardiovascular risk factor. The incidence of stroke and coronary heart disease in hypertensive patients who smoke is 2-3 times greater than in non-smoking patients with comparable blood pressure (*92*). Stopping smoking rapidly reduces this risk (*93*). Persuading hypertensive patients not to smoke is therefore the most effective single way a physician has to reduce their risk. Smoking control should also be an integral part of any programme for primary prevention of cardiovascular disease in populations.

Reduced fat intake. High serum cholesterol, high low-density lipoprotein-cholesterol, and low high-density lipoprotein-cholesterol levels increase the risk of atherosclerotic complications of hypertension, although there is some uncertainty whether this is true above the age of 70. Nutritional counselling and, when appropriate, drug treatment are indicated to control these risk factors. Hypertriglyceridaemia is a more debated cardiovascular risk factor, frequently associated with insulin-dependent and non-insulin-dependent diabetes mellitus and insulin-resistance. Increased physical activity and nutritional counselling are both recommended for treating hypertriglyceridaemia. Since increased physical activity is also likely to reduce body weight and blood pressure, it is most appropriate in hypertensive patients with hyperlipidaemia and disturbed glucose metabolism. Advice on nutrition and physical activity is an essential component of a primary prevention programme that aims to reduce the total risk of cardiovascular disease.

Control of diabetes. Diabetes requires a comprehensive plan of care which includes specific nutritional counselling and appropriate use of insulin and orally active hypoglycaemic drugs.

Several lifestyle measures (regular exercise, moderate weight reduction and a low-fat, high-carbohydrate, high-fibre diet) can improve insulin sensitivity and may help reduce the contribution of insulin resistance to increasing blood pressure.

Clinical trials of combined lifestyle changes. The effects of counselling to encourage reduction of dietary sodium and alcohol intake, weight loss and regular physical activity have been evaluated in various combinations in three clinical trials of primary prevention of hypertension in high-risk individuals. Hypertension incidence was reduced by 54% in the Primary Prevention of Hypertension study (*94*), by 20-35% in the Hypertension Prevention Trial (*95*), and by 51% with weight loss and 24% with sodium restriction in the Trials of Hypertension Prevention (*83*).

8.5 Health policy

Two complementary approaches have been proposed to control hypertension: the public health or population approach, and the clinical or individual approach (see section 8.1).

8.5.1 *Population approach*

Goals
The goals of the population approach are to:

- increase the population awareness that elevated blood pressure is a major health problem even though it may not be apparent
- help detect individuals who have hypertension or may be at risk of developing it
- advocate lifestyles which minimize if not eliminate the controllable risk factors of hypertension.

Components
To achieve the goals stated above, the population approach relies exclusively on educating the public, health professionals and patients with elevated blood pressure. The programme involves three key components.

1. Public education: the community must be informed about the nature, causes and complications of high blood pressure; its preventable and treatable nature; the lifestyle measures that are useful in its prevention and management; and the contributory role of other cardiovascular risk factors.

2. Professional education: physicians and other health professionals must be better trained to detect, manage and prevent high blood pressure. This requires appropriate emphasis in the curriculum as well as suitable training and certification procedures. The skills of health professionals to counsel individuals with high blood pressure and play an advocacy role in the community for the adoption of healthier lifestyles must be promoted.

3. Patient education: individuals with high blood pressure must be educated about their condition and its consequences, the need for effective management and the benefits of lifestyle changes. They also need to be told about the importance of adhering to health care advice (about lifestyle and, if appropriate, drug therapy) and the need for regular monitoring and periodic visits to the physician to discuss the effects of the therapy. The informed participation of family members must also be enlisted, while respecting the norms of medical confidentiality.

Methods of public education
Experience shows that there is no single way to educate the public for the simple reason that cultural, economic, environmental and geographical differences must be taken into consideration when developing the messages and deciding the most effective method of delivery.

Public announcements using radio, television, publications, community centres, work sites, schools and religious centres are important ways of communicating the message, but importance varies between countries. The message has to be simple, and repeated.

If successful, the population approach has been shown to have long-term effects (as in Canada, Finland and the United States of America). However, there are a number of requirements to achieve success:

– selecting the right approach for a given population
– developing a message that is culturally and socially acceptable
– recognizing the cost of such programmes
– evaluating the results (and cost) of the programme.

8.5.2 *Individual approach*

Although a population approach can have public health benefits, it is clear that many people with established hypertension may not respond sufficiently to non-pharmacological interventions. For these people, it is essential to develop an individual approach to treat hypertension. However, it is just as important to continue lifestyle modification as an adjunct to drug therapy.

8.5.3 *Components of a hypertension control policy*

Each country must develop a cogent health policy relevant to its identified needs based on lifestyle changes in the community as a whole and drug therapy in individuals with established high blood pressure. Components of such a policy may include:

— comprehensive health education programmes for communities including children;
— agricultural policies that help ensure that potassium-rich natural foods, like fresh fruit and vegetables, are readily available and inexpensive;
— regulation of the food industry to promote the availability of prepared food items with a low-salt and low-fat content, and labelling of marketed items for salt and fat content;
— providing facilities for outdoor recreational sports and leisure time;
— control of tobacco smoking which is an important additional risk factor for cardiovascular disease;
— ensuring the availability of inexpensive but effective drugs for lowering blood pressure;
— integration of programmes for blood pressure detection, treatment and control into the various levels of health care services, especially primary health care.

Most of these measures fit into an overall policy for health promotion aimed at controlling several lifestyle-related diseases. However, in specific instances, measures may be required which achieve the objectives of controlling high blood pressure without jeopardizing other public health objectives. For example, in countries where salt is used as a vehicle for iodine supplementation, alternative strategies for preventing iodine deficiency may need to be considered or the relative proportion of iodine to sodium chloride increased if feasible and safe. Planning and implementing programmes to control hypertension should involve health professionals, policy makers, and various governmental and non-governmental organizations. It is recommended that national and regional hypertension societies and leagues act in concert with health policy makers and health care providers to develop and deliver these programmes.

8.6 Research

8.6.1 *Epidemiological research*

Each country needs to develop an epidemiological database of:

— the distribution of blood pressure in different segments of the population
— the frequency of various factors contributing to the risk of developing high blood pressure
— the frequency of other cardiovascular risk factors that contribute to hypertension.

8.6.2 *Programme research*

Research is also needed in order to develop and implement control programmes appropriate to each level of health care and relevant to each community's needs.

8.6.3 *Evaluation research*

Blood pressure and risk factors should continue to be monitored and the cost–effectiveness of intervention programmes evaluated.

8.7 Implementation of population-based hypertension control programmes

National programmes to control high blood pressure are recommended in countries where hypertension has already been identified as a major health problem or where mean levels of blood pressure in the population are rising in parallel with lifestyle changes.

Every country should develop its own control programme based on the principles and guidelines given in this section. Programmes should be tailored to local needs and resources and, wherever possible, be established within the broader context of a comprehensive control programme for cardiovascular disease, as part of an integrated control programme for noncommunicable diseases.

Key elements of a programme should include:

— raising awareness of the problem among the community as a whole, health professionals, individuals with high blood pressure and policy makers
— advising/educating the community and individuals on how to promote and adopt healthy lifestyles, and the need for people with hypertension to adhere strictly to long-term therapeutic regimens
— ensuring active participation of all sectors of the community in the programme
— creating environmental conditions that support the adoption of healthy dietary and behaviour patterns (see section 8.5).

Each country should identify specific targets for prevention and treatment and specify the time period for their achievement. Progress should be monitored, and plans reviewed regularly.

9. Management of hypertension

In general, there is no identifiable cause for most patients with sustained arterial hypertension. If the cause is identified it should be treated in the appropriate manner, as described in section 5. Since treatment for hypertension is usually for life, the patient and the physician are committed to a long association. It is therefore important for the physician to establish effective communication with the patient, and take into account the patient's psychosocial status and preferences in arriving at a mutually agreed regimen of management. It is also important to integrate the treatment of the hypertension into an overall programme of management for associated risk factors and conditions, particularly in elderly patients who are more likely to have multiple associated disorders.

9.1 Goals of treatment

The goal of treatment should be the maximum tolerated reduction in blood pressure. Epidemiological studies show that, within the "normal" range of both systolic and diastolic blood pressures, the lower the blood pressure, the lower the risks of both stroke and coronary events (5). The safety of blood pressure reduction even at very low initial blood pressure levels has been indicated by the results of trials in patients with congestive heart failure or patients treated with ACE (angiotensin converting enzyme) inhibitors or β-blockers after myocardial infarction. Patients in the SHEP study (10) with an average initial DBP of 77 mmHg (10.3 kPa) exhibited substantial benefits with further lowering of blood pressure.

In mild hypertension, it would seem desirable in young patients (96) to achieve SBP of at least 120-130 mmHg (16.0-17.3 kPa) and DBP of 80 mmHg (10.7 kPa). In elderly patients it would seem desirable to lower blood pressure to below 140 mmHg (18.7 kPa) for SBP and 90 mmHg (12.0 kPa) for DBP, while in patients with isolated systolic hypertension the goal should be SBP of at least 140 mmHg (18.7 kPa) if this is tolerated. Blood pressure measurements by ambulatory methods are on average several mmHg lower than clinic blood pressure (18); therefore, goals for blood pressure assessed by these techniques should be set at a lower level to avoid undertreatment.

9.2 Lifestyle measures

Lifestyle measures (non-pharmacological treatments) are used for four complementary reasons:

— to lower blood pressure in the individual patient
— to reduce the need for antihypertensive drugs
— to minimize associated risk factors in an individual
— primary prevention of hypertension and associated cardiovascular diseases in populations.

Since they can reduce the overall risk of cardiovascular disease as well as lower blood pressure, lifestyle measures should be applied before considering drug treatment, especially in patients with mild hypertension, and should form an integral component of the overall management programme for all hypertensive patients. Since lifestyle measures are discussed extensively in sections 3 and 8 they will only be listed here.

Table 10
Guidelines for selecting first-line drugs for hypertension

Class of drug	Condition/indications	Contraindications	Caution/limited value
Diuretics	Heart failure Elderly patients Systolic hypertension Black patients	Gout	Diabetes Hyperlipidaemia Pregnancy[a] Sexually active males
β-Blockers	Angina After myocardial infarct Tachyarrhythmias Pregnancy	Asthma and chronic obstructive pulmonary disease Peripheral vascular disease Heart block[b]	Hypertriglyceridaemia Insulin-dependent diabetes mellitus Heart failure Athletes and physically active patients Black patients
ACE inhibitors	Heart failure Left ventricular hypertrophy After myocardial infarct Diabetes with micro-albuminuria	Pregnancy Bilateral renal artery stenosis	Black patients
Calcium antagonists	Angina Peripheral vascular disease Elderly patients Systolic hypertension Glucose intolerance Black patients	Pregnancy	Congestive heart failure[c] Atrioventricular heart block[d]
α-Blockers	Prostatic hypertrophy Glucose intolerance		Orthostatic hypotension

[a] Because of reduced plasma volume.
[b] Grade II and III atrioventricular block.
[c] Verapamil should be avoided or used only with great caution.
[d] Verapamil and diltiazem should be avoided or used only with great caution.

Lifestyle measures that contribute to lowering blood pressure:

- weight reduction
- reduction of alcohol intake
- increased physical activity
- moderation of dietary sodium.

Lifestyle measures for the treatment of associated risk factors:

- cessation of tobacco smoking
- reduced fat intake
- control of diabetes.

9.3 Drug treatment

There is general agreement that five classes of drug are most suitable for the first-line treatment of patients with hypertension (*12, 13*): diuretics, β-blockers, ACE inhibitors, calcium antagonists and α-blockers (Table 10). Other classes of drug may be used in certain situations.

9.3.1 *Diuretics*

Diuretics have been widely used as first-line antihypertensive therapy, and have been shown to prevent cardiovascular morbidity and mortality, especially fatal and non-fatal stroke (*9*). Particularly in large doses, diuretics may cause a variety of unwanted metabolic effects – principally potassium depletion, reduced glucose tolerance (*97*), ventricular ectopic beats and impotence (*92*). These can be reduced by keeping the dose as low as possible. Low-dose diuretics remain effective, not only in lowering elevated blood pressure, but in reducing cardiovascular morbidity and mortality, as shown in recent trials in elderly patients (*10, 11, 14, 15*). Diuretics are also inexpensive. They are particularly valuable as ancillary treatment to enhance the effectiveness of many other types of antihypertensive drug. A combination of diuretics with potassium-sparing drugs or with ACE inhibitors may prevent potassium depletion.

9.3.2 *β-Blockers*

β-Adrenoceptor-blocking drugs (β-blockers) are safe, cheap and effective. They are widely used in subjects of all ages with hypertension of all degrees of severity. They have been part of the treatment regimen in many of the major studies that have demonstrated reduction in morbidity and mortality attributable to lowering blood pressure (*9*).

A large variety of β-blockers is available. Some are cardio-selective, while others demonstrate some intrinsic sympathomimetic activity or have α-blocking or vasodilator properties (*12, 13*). Although β-blockers have been shown to be useful in the secondary prevention of myocardial infarction (*98*), they have not been shown to have any advantage over diuretics in the primary prevention of myocardial infarction in hypertensive patients (*12*).

9.3.3 *ACE inhibitors*

ACE inhibitors have been demonstrated to be safe and effective in lowering blood pressure. They are well tolerated by most patients and do not have any metabolic side effects. The most common adverse effect is a dry, persistent cough; a very rare, though serious, side effect is angio-oedema. ACE inhibitors should be prescribed in low doses to patients with impaired renal function, and should be avoided in patients with bilateral stenosis of the renal arteries (*12, 13*). ACE inhibitors should generally be avoided in pregnancy; they are strongly contraindicated in the second half of pregnancy since they may cause fetal and neonatal death (*99*).

ACE inhibitors have not yet been shown to decrease cardiovascular morbidity and mortality in hypertensive patients (*12, 13*). However, they have been shown to reduce morbidity and mortality, including from coronary events, in patients with congestive heart failure and after myocardial infarction in patients with reduced ejection fraction (*100, 101*) by mitigating left ventricular dilation (*101*). ACE inhibitors have also been shown to be very effective in reducing the development of left ventricular hypertrophy in hypertensive patients (*102*), and retarding the progression of renal disease in patients with insulin-dependent diabetes mellitus and moderate renal impairment (*103*).

9.3.4 *Calcium antagonists*

There are three major groups of calcium antagonists with distinctly different properties: the phenylalkylamines (verapamil), dihydropyridines (nifedipine) and benzothiazepines (diltiazem). Calcium antagonists are safe and effective in lowering blood pressure (*12, 13*). Side effects include tachycardia, headache and flushing (especially with the fast-acting dihydropyridines), ankle oedema and constipation (with verapamil). Calcium antagonists do not appear to have adverse metabolic effects, but their safety profile has not yet been established in early pregnancy (*12, 13*). There is so far no evidence from long-term trials that calcium antagonists can lower morbidity or mortality in hypertension (*12, 13*).

9.3.5 *α-Blockers*

α-Adrenoceptor-blocking drugs (α-blockers) are safe and effective in lowering blood pressure (*12, 13*). The main side effect is postural hypotension which may be seen after the first dose and which can be a particular problem in elderly patients and in patients with autonomic neuropathy (*12, 13*). Assessment of blood pressure when the patient is standing is essential when using α-blockers (*13*). There is some evidence that α-blockers may have advantages in patients with hyperlipidaemia or glucose intolerance (*12*). As with the other newer agents, there are no long-term clinical trials demonstrating reduction in morbidity or mortality in hypertensive patients treated with α-blockers (*12, 13*).

9.3.6 *Other classes of drug*

Drugs acting on the central nervous system are also effective anti-hypertensive agents and have been used for many years. They have been used in several controlled clinical trials, mostly in association with diuretics, that have proved the ability of antihypertensive therapy to reduce cardiovascular events (9). In particular, methyldopa remains an important, well-validated agent for the effective treatment of hyper-tension in pregnancy (*12, 13*). Although relatively cheap, centrally acting drugs have worse side effects than the antihypertensive agents previously mentioned. If centrally acting drugs, such as reserpine, are used in low-income populations because of their cost–effectiveness, it is recommended that they be used in combination with diuretics and prescribed in much lower doses than in earlier years.

Direct vasodilators, such as hydralazine and minoxidil, are also quite effective in lowering blood pressure, but some of their side effects (tachycardia, headache and sodium and water retention) make it difficult to use them as monotherapy.

9.3.7 *Combination of drugs*

If a drug from any of the five major pharmacological classes is ineffective in lowering blood pressure in a given patient, it is reasonable to substitute a drug from a different class. If therapy with a single drug is only partly effective, it may be preferable to add a small dose of a second drug from another class rather than increase the dose (*104*). This permits the addition of different primary actions while minimizing the homoeostatic compensations that limit the fall in pressure (*104*). Combination therapy also minimizes side effects by encouraging the use of drugs in low doses.

An additive effect has been shown when combining:

- a diuretic with a β-blocker, ACE inhibitor or α-blocker
- a β-blocker with an α-blocker or a dihydropyridine calcium antagonist
- an ACE inhibitor with a calcium antagonist.

In order to maximize the benefits of treatment in all hypertensive patients, combinations of two and sometimes three drugs may be required.

For reasons of convenience, cost and increased patient compliance, preparations that combine two drugs in a single tablet or capsule may be appropriate for many patients once the need and dose for constituent drugs have been established.

9.4   Combination of drug treatment and lifestyle measures

A number of treatment trials have indicated the ability of lifestyle changes – weight reduction (*105*), potassium increase (*106*) and sodium restriction (*107*) – to maintain blood pressure control with lower doses of antihypertensive drugs. The TOMHS Study indicates the additive benefit of lifestyle changes combined with a low dose of any one drug from each of the five classes of first-line drugs (*107*). One unexpected finding in a number of studies has been that the combination of drug and non-drug treatment produced a reduction in adverse effects and an improved quality of life compared with lifestyle change or drug treatment alone (*104, 105, 107, 108*). There is also some limited data suggesting that combined treatment provides even greater reduction in cardiovascular risk (*108, 109*).

9.5 Management plan

9.5.1 *"Mild" hypertension*

The decision to treat should be based not only on the diastolic and systolic blood pressures but on the total cardiovascular risk in the individual patient (see Table 1). With moderate and severe hypertension, SBP greater than 180 mmHg (24.0 kPa) and DBP greater than 105 mmHg (14.0 kPa), treatment should be initiated without delay, even in the absence of other risk factors or conditions. However, with mild hypertension, SBP 140-180 mmHg (18.7-24.0 kPa) or DBP 90-105 mmHg (12.0-14.0 kPa), the decision to treat should be taken only after careful initial assessment over a period of weeks or months, as illustrated in Fig. 3.

In practice, when the initial SBP is 140-180 mmHg (18.7-24.0 kPa) or DBP is 90-105 mmHg (12.0-14.0 kPa), measurements should be repeated on at least two further occasions during the next four weeks before labelling a subject as hypertensive and deciding to initiate treatment. This is particularly important as both systolic and diastolic pressures are subject to natural variation.

All patients should be advised to modify their lifestyle, as appropriate, by stopping smoking, reducing obesity, limiting alcohol and dietary saturated fat, restricting salt intake and engaging in regular, mild dynamic exercise. This advice should form a very important part of the strategies to reduce blood pressure and to improve cardiovascular health. Management decisions should be made after discussion with the patient and his/her family and outlining the risks and benefits of various intervention strategies.

Practical guidelines for management are illustrated in Fig. 3.

If the blood pressure falls below 140 mmHg (18.7 kPa) SBP and 90 mmHg (12.0 kPa) DBP within four weeks, it should be monitored at three-monthly intervals for a year, and then annually.

If within four weeks the blood pressure remains in the range 140-180 mmHg (18.7-24.0 kPa) SBP or 90-105 mmHg (12.0-14.0 kPa) DBP and the total cardiovascular risk is high (especially if there is evidence of target organ damage), lifestyle measures should be re-inforced and drug treatment initiated. If the total cardiovascular risk is

Figure 3
Management plan for mild hypertension[a]

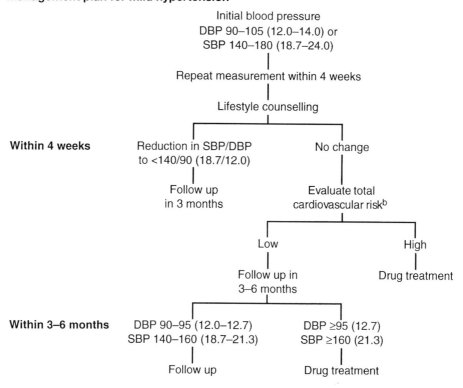

WHO 96017

[a] Blood pressure shown in mmHg (kPa).
[b] If target organ damage is present, drug treatment is necessary at any level of mild hypertension, i.e. SBP 140-180 mmHg (18.7-24.0 kPa) or DBP 90-105 mmHg (12.0-14.0 kPa).

low and there are no signs of target organ damage, lifestyle measures should be reinforced and blood pressure monitored for 3-6 months, depending on the level of the blood pressure.

After 3-6 months, if blood pressure is 140-160 mmHg (18.7-21.3 kPa) SBP or 90-95 mmHg (12.0-12.7 kPa) DBP but there are no other cardiovascular risk factors present, lifestyle measures and blood pressure monitoring should continue. However if the blood pressure is still above or equal to 160 mmHg (21.3 kPa) SBP or 95 mmHg (12.7 kPa) DBP, drug treatment should be instituted.

Choice of drugs in patients with mild hypertension
Of the five classes of first-line drugs, only diuretics and β-blockers have been used in long-term studies demonstrating that lowering blood pressure reduces morbidity and mortality (9). However, it is important to note that all these studies were designed to demonstrate the benefits of

lowering blood pressure *per se* rather than the benefits of a specific drug or class of drug (9). The success of diuretics and β-blockers in establishing the reduction in cardiovascular morbidity and mortality with reduced blood pressure is important since it has validated the extrapolation of the benefits to other individual drugs within a particular class of drugs, to other classes of drugs and to lifestyle measures effective in lowering blood pressure.

The choice of antihypertensive drugs will depend on socioeconomic factors that determine availability in different countries or regions and the characteristics of the individual patient, particularly the presence of risk factors for cardiovascular disease, target organ damage and coexisting disorders and possible side effects. The particular advantages and disadvantages of the various classes of drug are described above and summarized in Table 10.

There are not yet many studies on the comparative efficacy of different classes of drug in lowering systolic pressure in elderly subjects with isolated systolic hypertension.

9.5.2 *Moderate and severe hypertension*

Patients presenting with average DBP of 105–120 mmHg (14.0–16.0 kPa) and/or SBP of 180–210 mmHg (24.0–28.0 kPa) should be referred for immediate evaluation and assessed carefully for target organ damage, associated cardiovascular risk factors and history of previous antihypertensive therapy. Drug therapy should not be delayed in patients with target organ damage or with multiple risk factors. Patients should be seen after two weeks of active therapy. If the fall in blood pressure is inadequate, a second drug from a different pharmacological class should be added and blood pressure measured at frequent intervals. Lifestyle measures and patient education are equally important in this group.

Patients with DBP averaging more than 120 mmHg and/or SBP greater than 210 mmHg (28.0 kPa) require immediate drug therapy while they undergo laboratory evaluation. Most of these patients require more than one drug in order to control their hypertension. The severity of the hypertension and the presence of complications will determine the intensity of antihypertensive treatment and the frequency of observation.

Most of the antihypertensive drugs when given orally require a period of 3–6 weeks to achieve a maximal antihypertensive effect. Some calcium antagonists, ACE inhibitors, β-blockers, centrally acting drugs and loop diuretics can produce rapid lowering of blood pressure when given orally.

9.5.3 *Resistant hypertension*

Patients who continue to have moderate to severe high blood pressure after therapy with three or more drugs for at least one month have resistant hypertension. Causes of resistance include lack of patient compliance, inadequate drug dosage, inappropriate drug combinations, expansion of blood volume, use of pressor medications and the presence of secondary forms of hypertension. Excess salt and alcohol intake are other causes of resistance to therapy; and the "white coat effect" (where a patient's blood pressure only becomes elevated in the presence of a doctor or a nurse) can cause apparent resistance. Expansion of blood volume secondary to lowering of blood pressure, intrinsic renal disease and side effects of drugs are very important causes of resistance to treatment. Use of loop diuretics in large doses can help to bring resistant hypertension under control in some patients. The combination of ACE inhibitors and calcium antagonists has proved to be especially effective in severe and resistant cases (13). Patients with resistant hypertension require extended evaluation.

9.5.4 *Hypertensive emergencies*

The following conditions need rapid reduction of blood pressure and require admittance to hospital with immediate intervention: severe hypertension with papilloedema or haemorrhages in the optic fundus (malignant and accelerated hypertension), hypertension complicated by acute left ventricular failure, cerebrovascular accident, acute coronary event, acute aortic dissection, hypertensive encephalopathy, hypertensive crisis of phaeochromocytoma, eclampsia, and hypertension following cardiac surgery or due to a food or drug interaction with a monoamine oxidase inhibitor. There are a number of therapeutic options for hypertensive emergencies (13). The choice depends upon the clinical situation and the experience of the physician. Drugs used include intravenous furosemide, sublingual or intravenous infusion of nitroglycerin, or nifedipine capsules chewed and swallowed. In situations where immediate reduction of blood pressure is necessary, intravenous infusion with sodium nitroprusside, an intravenous bolus or infusion of diazoxide, and intravenous labetalol are very effective. In the hypertensive crisis of phaeochromocytoma, phentolamine should be administered.

9.6 Follow-up procedures

During the stabilization period of treatment, patients need to be seen at regular intervals until blood pressure levels are satisfactorily controlled. The main task of doctors during follow up is to ensure that the target systolic and diastolic blood pressure is reached and maintained and that other risk factors are controlled. Gradual and careful lowering of blood pressure will minimize side effects and complications of treatment, and improve compliance. Sometimes telling a patient that he or she has hypertension ("labelling") may be followed by anxiety or mood changes. Reassurance about the prognosis and his or her ability to lead a normal active life is therefore particularly important, as is the need to explain any new symptoms that may appear. Self-measurement of blood pressure may be helpful to ensure compliance. After stabilization of blood pressure, follow-up visits at 3–6 month intervals may be adequate.

As a rule, antihypertensive therapy should be maintained indefinitely. Cessation of therapy in patients who had been correctly diagnosed as having hypertension is usually followed – sooner or later – by return of blood pressure to pretreatment levels. Nevertheless, after prolonged blood pressure control it may be possible to attempt a careful progressive reduction in the dose or number of drugs used, especially in patients strictly adhering to lifestyle changes. Attempts to step down the treatment should be accompanied, however, by careful, continued supervision of blood pressure.

9.7 Communicating with hypertensive patients

Communication should be a two-way process in which health worker and patient listen to each other and exchange information. The purpose is for the health worker to find out about the patient in order to be able to provide appropriate information on his or her condition and subsequent treatment. Such patient education is an important component of health care in general, and of care of hypertensive patients in particular.

Effective communication requires special skills which physicians and allied health personnel do not always possess or realize the importance of mastering. Communication and counselling skills should therefore be included in the curricula of all health professions, especially in view of the need to respect patient autonomy.

9.7.1 *One-to-one communication*

The implications for the patient of being diagnosed as hypertensive, the prognosis and the advantages of medical care need to be carefully communicated at the first meeting with the physician. The patient's preferences regarding drug or non-pharmacological treatment can be explored at this early stage; this may help to understand the patient better and to win his or her cooperation to comply to a treatment programme. Using a combination of instructions and dialogue (*110*), the physician should guide the patient on ways to control his or her blood pressure and associated risk factors if present. Compliance with a recommended therapeutic/preventive regimen is a long-term, even permanent issue, requiring ongoing educational efforts on the part of the physician or health worker.

One special task of the communication/education process is to identify and correct the patient's misconceptions regarding hypertension (e.g. that treatment is necessary only when the patient has a headache or feels dizzy). A number of skills, such as mnemonic techniques for remembering to take drugs, or self-measurement of blood pressure, may be part of the education process.

9.7.2 *Group education*

One-to-one communication/education can be extended to group education. Certain patients may need the reinforcement that a group can provide in order to implement changes in lifestyle. Other patients may require an advanced degree of instruction to address particularly difficult behavioural modifications, such as stopping smoking and controlling obesity.

Patients with strong social support tend to adhere better to recommended antihypertensive therapy, and for this reason it is useful to include spouses and other family members in the education programme. Children can be particularly helpful in promoting healthy lifestyles by increasing the motivation of a parent. Health promotion programmes in schools can provide children with the information they need to fulfil this role.

10. Cost–effectiveness

The cost-effectiveness of managing hypertension is the balance between benefits and costs. Benefits include the prevention of morbid and fatal cardiovascular and renal events, and the improvement in the quality of life gained by avoiding admission to hospital, the need for rehabilitation and the possibility of functional sequelae. These benefits are obtained at the financial cost of visits to the physician, supplementary examinations, drugs and management of adverse effects related to treatment, in addition to the qualitative cost of changes in lifestyle. Formal cost-effectiveness analyses have been performed and provide a theoretical basis for optimizing diagnosis and treatment strategies (*111-114*).

The successful management of hypertension should be evaluated not only by the achievement of medical goals, such as blood pressure control and correction of cardiovascular risk factors, but also by the appropriateness of the resources used (*115*). The cost-effectiveness of the management of hypertension should be optimal for the individual and the community.

10.1 The individual approach

Resources are used in all aspects of the investigation and management of the hypertensive patient.

10.1.1 *Diagnosis*

The diagnostic process includes many clinical, biological, imaging and genetic methods. However, there are inequalities between social groups and countries in accessing these methods. In order to make the management of hypertension cost-effective, certain general rules should be applied to the diagnostic process.

1. Examinations should be ranked according to their simplicity, feasibility, safety and cost. Priority should be given to carrying out a complete clinical examination to a high standard.

2. A test should be selected only if its significance for the decision-making process has been demonstrated.

3. Even when highly specific and highly sensitive, a diagnostic test is worth while only if the prevalence of the particular condition in a given medical context is sufficiently high.

4. Calibration of devices used to measure blood pressure as well as measurement of the observer's performance should ensure the accuracy, precision, reproducibility, and validity of an examination.

These general rules apply to different methods of blood pressure measurement, as well as to echocardiography, ultrasound and radiological examinations, and biochemical and genetic investigations.

The diversity of the clinical patterns of hypertension and the introduction of new diagnostic techniques make the selection of appropriate supplementary examinations for a given individual more and more complex. In order to avoid unjustified expense, this selection needs to be guided by the available evidence of quality of the tests and their expected influence on the decision-making process.

10.1.2 *Treatment*

The increasing number of antihypertensive drugs means that physicians can tailor therapy to meet the needs of individual patients. The diversity of hypertensive patients, cardiovascular risk factors and concomitant diseases (especially in the elderly) and the occurrence of various early or late side effects makes it impossible to opt for a single rigid and standardized therapeutic schedule.

The cost of drugs always represents a large part of the overall cost of hypertension management. Ensuring the cost–effective use of drugs through drug pricing and reimbursement mechanisms is the joint responsibility of manufacturers, suppliers, prescribers and health authorities. In countries where national resources do not restrict access to drugs, everyone should have equal access to all drugs for which efficacy, tolerability and safety have been documented; preference should be given to those drugs with proven superiority in terms of control of blood pressure, improved quality of life, regression of target organ damage, and decreased morbidity and mortality. For countries in which access to care is constrained by economic factors, simplified strategies are needed, with emphasis on efficacy, safety and costs as guided by the "essential" drugs listed by WHO (*116*).

10.2 The population approach

The cost-effectiveness of detection and care of hypertension depends on individual countries adjusting action programmes to suit their health care systems and the blood-pressure-related characteristics of their populations. Which approach will be the most cost-effective depends on factors such as the number of physicians per inhabitant and the availability of community medicine, family medicine and occupational medicine.

Certain general rules are valid for the population approach in all countries in the same way as they are for the practice of clinical medicine. Screening is useless in the absence of appropriate follow up. Multiplication of competing health care systems within a particular country may lead to inefficiency. Selective efforts for detecting and managing hypertension may be more cost-effective within broader programmes of preventive medicine. The cost-effectiveness of structured programmes for implementing patient education and lifestyle changes should also be evaluated.

The modification of lifestyle, including nutritional habits, should be tailored to the characteristics of each community. Prevention of some risk factors such as alcohol abuse and dependence, smoking and obesity may be the most cost-effective because of their impact on events other than cardiovascular diseases, such as traffic accidents, lung cancer, chronic bronchitis and arthrosis.

10.3 Ethical aspects of cost–effectiveness

The management of hypertension is based on minimizing the absolute risk of all hypertensive individuals. However, the perception of the absolute risk and of the benefits and costs of its reduction varies from one individual to another. Treatment will be more costly and require more active participation for some patients than for others, and some may disagree with the advice they are given. It is therefore important to find out the patient's preferences when deciding the treatment programme to ensure adherence and increase cost-effectiveness.

On the other hand, at the population level, resources might be used more effectively in the fight against other more urgent health problems. However, such a choice should only be considered as temporary, the ultimate goal being to provide hypertensive patients all over the world the same access to, and the same quality of, care. This objective is worth while in low-income economies, and in high-income economies where the deleterious influence of hypertension on cardiovascular health has been shown to be particularly marked in economically disadvantaged communities with high unemployment and low levels of education. Ethically, cost-effectiveness of hypertension management can only be judged at the global level.

11. Evaluation of hypertension control in populations

In many communities and/or countries significant efforts and resources have been directed to the control of hypertension.

11.1 Rationale

There are at least three reasons to evaluate the status of hypertension control in populations. First, there is a strategic need, i.e. the need to find out whether the various aspects of control policies are adequate, and how they could be improved. Secondly, there are economic reasons for evaluating the cost–effectiveness of existing policies because community programmes for hypertension may draw resources away from other, perhaps more significant programmes. Thirdly, there are strong ethical reasons for monitoring how hypertension control is being carried out, what kind of influence existing programmes have on the health status of communities, and whether they have side effects at the population level.

This section discusses possible measures and/or indices to assess whether population-based interventions result in positive public health outcomes. Evaluating the outcome of hypertension control is difficult. Although it is tempting to look solely at changes in death rates from hypertension complications, this is not a true indication because there is not a direct relation between these death rates and hypertension control. For example, in the United States of America mortality from stroke began to decline long before the discovery of antihypertensive agents. On the other hand, the rate of this decline accelerated shortly after the inception of the National High Blood Pressure Education Program.

Few evaluations of hypertension control in populations have been formally and scientifically conducted and/or reported. In the WHO-coordinated study on the community control of hypertension, "intervention" and "reference" communities were compared (*117*). Blood pressure values, awareness of hypertension (i.e. whether subjects had been told that their blood pressure was elevated) and rates of treated and untreated hypertensive individuals were assessed. Results showed that in both "intervention" and "reference" communities there was a decrease in high blood pressure values and an increase in the rates of awareness and of treatment.

11.2 Hypertension management audit

In the Hypertension Management Audit Project conducted by the World Health Organization's Regional Office for Europe and the World Hypertension League (*118, 119*), the following approaches were used to assess the control of hypertension in participating European communities.

1. The "population approach" consisted of a classical, epidemiological survey of a random sample of a population. Its aims were to assess the basic indicators of awareness of hypertension in the community, such as the proportion of undiagnosed and untreated, as well as over-diagnosed and possibly unnecessarily treated, hypertensive patients.

2. In the "patient approach", a sample of patients with established hypertension was selected, and their case histories were reviewed by a small committee of investigators. This patient survey was a medical audit in the strict sense of the term – a retrospective assessment of the quality of care on the basis of medical records, combined with re-examinations of the patient. The WHO/ISH (International Society of Hypertension) guidelines for the management of mild hypertension were selected as the standard of adequate treatment, with which the actual management of the audited patients was compared.

3. In the "consumer approach", patients are the consumers of medical care. Their perceptions and satisfaction were taken as important indicators of certain aspects of the complex process of hypertension control. The consumer inquiry was an attempt to assess the clients, mood, their readiness to follow advice, and their possible complaints about the care received.

4. The "physician approach" consisted of an inquiry to assess the knowledge and attitudes of physicians involved in the control of hypertension. To this effect, a questionnaire was addressed to a sample of general practitioners and specialists in internal medicine. The replies were limited to knowledge and attitudes. In all likelihood they did not measure what physicians are in fact doing, but described rather what they thought they ought to do. Still, these "self portraits" are valuable in the sense that actual behaviour is unlikely to be better than the ideas and intentions of the respondents.

5. The "drug utilization approach" used established methods to assess the volume of antihypertensive drugs prescribed in defined daily doses, related to the number of inhabitants of a community and the prevalence of hypertension. It also assessed the pattern of drug utilization. Both amount and structure are valuable health-care indices, which may complement the information received from the epidemiological and clinical approaches.

This five-step approach to evaluation has produced a great number of relevant indicators of the quality of antihypertensive management. These are the degree of awareness of hypertension in the population, the percentage of missed appointments, the attitudes of physicians to therapy and the pattern of drug prescribing. The project is one of the first to report on patients' satisfaction with the therapy used to manage hypertension. The varied results indicate that more attention should be paid to this component of hypertension management. Physicians need more formal training in this domain. This project has also shown, however, that new methods are needed to influence physicians' acceptance of and compliance with recommendations for the diagnosis and management of hypertensive patients.

11.3 Time trends

In the United States of America the effectiveness of the population-based programme has been evaluated repeatedly by means of surveys measuring the number of people diagnosed as having hypertension, the number undergoing treatment and the number whose blood pressure is under control. The results from these successive surveys are shown in Table 11.

The changes shown in Table 11, plus the accelerated decline in death rate from stroke and coronary heart disease during the same period of time, support the effectiveness of population-based interventions in the United States of America (*120*).

There are many other databases that could be used to assess the status of hypertension control in populations; for example data from the WHO MONICA Project (*33*) which monitors the major risk factors of coronary heart disease and stroke in men and women aged 35–64 years in over 40 populations. Routinely available information on morbidity, such as the proportion of stroke patients with controlled and uncontrolled hypertension before the attack, could also be used.

Table 11
Rates of hypertension[a] awareness, treatment and control in the United States of America

	Percentage of population[b]			
Category	1971–1972	1974–1975	1976–1980	1988–1991
Aware: told by physician that they have hypertension	51	64	73 (54)	84 (65)
Treated: taking medication	36	34	56 (33)	73 (49)
Controlled: SBP/DBP <160/95 mmHg (21.3/12.7 kPa) on one occasion and taking antihypertensive medication	16	20	34 (11)	55 (21)

[a] Defined as SBP/DBP of 160/95 mmHg (21.3/21.7 kPa) or more on one occasion or reported to be taking antihypertensive medication. Numbers in parentheses indicate the percentage of the population with SBP/DBP at 140/90 mmHg (18.7/12.0 kPa) or more.
[b] Source: unpublished data provided by the Centers for Disease Control and Prevention, National Center for Health Statistics, Atlanta, GA, USA:
1971–1972 and 1974–1975 – National Health and Nutrition Examination Survey I
1976–1980 – National Health and Nutrition Examination Survey II
1988–1991 – National Health and Nutrition Examination Survey III

11.4 Cost of evaluation

Although resources are needed to evaluate the process and the outcome of hypertension control, the cost is estimated to be only a small fraction of the overall cost of hypertension control in a population. It is essential, however, that the information obtained from evaluation is used properly to improve hypertension control in respective populations.

12. Conclusions and recommendations

12.1 Overview

Hypertension is a massive health problem affecting about 20% of the adult population in most countries. It is one of the major risk factors for cardiovascular mortality, which accounts for 20–50% of all deaths, and for morbidity, which contributes to disability and health care costs.

The WHO Expert Committee recommends that a major long-term goal for all countries should be to eliminate preventable cardiovascular diseases in the young and middle-aged, and to reduce them markedly in the elderly. To achieve this the Expert Committee recommends that control programmes for hypertension be set up as part of a comprehensive strategy for the reduction of total cardiovascular risk. Such strategies should also address other major risk factors for cardiovascular disease: smoking, raised serum cholesterol and diabetes.

The Committee believes that the primary prevention of hypertension is critically important for attaining these long-term goals, and has described the measures that should be implemented for this purpose.

The success of these strategies will depend on increased financial and human resources being allocated to their implementation and evaluation.

The present report outlines the existing state of knowledge of hypertension, and makes suggestions for a population approach to prevention and control in countries with various resources and health care systems. It also outlines current approaches to the assessment and management of the individual patient, and identifies areas for further research into hypertension control.

12.2 Conclusions

1. Blood pressure values are normally distributed in populations and there is a continuum of increasing cardiovascular risk associated with increasing levels of both systolic and diastolic blood pressure. There is no dividing line between normotension and hypertension, but a practical definition of hypertension can be made on the basis of intervention trials that have identified the pressures at which reduction results in significant benefits.

2. The definition and classification of the degree of hypertension provide a simple and reliable method of assessing an individual patient's total cardiovascular risk in order to determine appropriate treatment. Classification allows assessment of the level of risk associated with raised blood pressure, but also takes into consideration the other risk factors such as smoking, dyslipidaemia, glucose intolerance and diabetes, and development of hypertension-related organ damage.

3. Adults with systolic blood pressure of 140 mmHg (18.7 kPa) or above or a level of diastolic pressure of 90 mmHg (12.0 kPa) or above should be defined as being hypertensive. Those whose blood pressures are in the range of 140–160 mmHg (18.7–21.3 kPa) for systolic values and 90–95 mmHg (12.0–12.7 kPa) for diastolic values should be defined as borderline hypertensive as the associated risk of cardiovascular disease is rather low; however, they may benefit from treatment if the level of other risk factors is high.

4. The terms "mild", "moderate" and "severe" hypertension have been retained because of their common use in the clinical setting. It should be emphasized that, as currently used, these terms refer simply to the extent of the blood pressure elevation. The severity of the clinical condition depends on the total cardiovascular risk of the patient and, in particular, on associated organ damage. Accordingly the classification of hypertension based on three stages of organ damage put forward in the 1978 Expert Committee report is retained (see Table 3, page 9).

5. Untreated hypertension increases the risk of vascular damage involving both small arteries and arterioles, and large arteries. These lesions lead to coronary heart disease, congestive heart failure, stroke and renal dysfunction. Concurrence of other risk factors, such as smoking, raised serum cholesterol and diabetes, will augment and accelerate organ damage and may also influence the type of lesion incurred.

6. The diagnostic programme for a patient in whom high blood pressure has been found should be directed to several goals:

    – confirming a chronic elevation of blood pressure
    – assessing the total cardiovascular risk
    – evaluating existing organ damage or concomitant disease
    – searching for possible causes of the hypertension.

    A detailed medical history and physical examination will help to indicate the laboratory investigations needed. Simple tests are satisfactory in diagnosing mild to moderate hypertension in the majority of patients; progressively more detailed tests are needed for severe and complicated hypertension.

7. An accurate assessment of blood pressure is essential. This is usually done in the clinic or physician's office with a mercury manometer

by the auscultatory method, with the patient resting in the seated position. The physician's (or nurse's) assessment can also be complemented by blood pressure measurements taken at home by the patient or a relative, provided they are suitably trained. Twenty-four-hour monitoring of ambulatory blood pressure can also be useful in a few specific situations. Whenever measurements made at home or by ambulatory blood pressure monitoring are used for clinical decisions, it should be remembered that blood pressure values provided by these techniques are on average several mmHg lower than levels measured in a clinic. Blood pressure thresholds for diagnosing hypertension and for defining treatment goals should be set at a lower level when assessed by these techniques to avoid underdiagnosis and undertreatment.

8. The use of the term "white-coat hypertension" to indicate blood pressure that is raised only when measured in a clinical setting could be replaced by the term "isolated clinic hypertension". The prognostic implication of this phenomenon has not yet been elucidated.

9. In some women estrogen–progestogen oral contraceptives can cause marked elevation of blood pressure. It is not known whether hormonal contraceptives with a low estrogen content or containing only progestogen cause a similar rise in blood pressure. On the other hand, there is no contraindication on blood-pressure grounds to the use of hormone replacement therapy with low-dose estrogen in post-menopausal women, but blood pressure should be monitored more frequently.

10. The hypertensive disease of pregnancy is a major cause of premature birth and perinatal death and is also responsible for 20–33% of all maternal deaths. It is a major health problem in developing countries.

11. In most populations blood pressure increases progressively with age. The rate of rise appears to be influenced by the levels of blood pressure in childhood or early adult life ("tracking"), ethnicity and sex. The absence of an age-related rise in some populations suggests that lifestyle factors such as diet and exercise are also important determinants of the relation between blood pressure and age.

12. Hypertension is more common in people aged 65 years or more, among whom isolated systolic hypertension is particularly frequent. In absolute terms, hypertension is a much greater risk factor for cardiovascular events in the elderly than in young people; correspondingly, numerous intervention trials have shown that the absolute benefit of antihypertensive therapy, even in isolated systolic hypertension, is particularly high in the elderly. Efforts should be made to avoid sudden drops in blood pressure and orthostatic hypotension in elderly patients. Low-dose medication is often successful. Concomitant disease, frequent in the elderly, should influence the decision to treat and the mode of treatment.

13. Non-insulin-dependent diabetes mellitus is two to three times as frequent in hypertensive populations as in non-hypertensive populations. Patients with hypertension and diabetes mellitus are especially vulnerable to cardiovascular and renal complications; therefore, the control of hypertension and dyslipidaemia, as well as cessation of smoking, are particularly important.

14. The risk of developing hypertension is influenced by heredity, and a positive family history is a strong risk factor. Hypertension, for the most part, is currently regarded as a polygenic disorder. Specific gene disorders are under investigation and some have already been described.

15. Excess body weight, low levels of physical activity and excess consumption of salt or alcohol are important lifestyle factors contributing to the development of high blood pressure. Dietary potassium may be protective.

16. Observational cohort studies suggest that lower blood pressure values are associated with a substantially lower incidence of major complications. This has been confirmed by intervention studies.

17. Of the five classes of first-line drugs, only diuretics and β-blockers have been used in long-term studies demonstrating that lowering blood pressure reduces morbidity and mortality. However, all these studies were designed to demonstrate the benefits of lowering blood pressure *per se* rather than the benefits of a specific drug or class of drugs. The success of certain diuretics and β-blockers in reducing cardiovascular morbidity and mortality by lowering blood pressure is critically important since it has validated the extrapolation of the benefits to other drugs within the same two classes, to other classes of drugs and to the lifestyle measures that are effective in lowering blood pressure.

18. Combinations of two or more drugs from different classes are necessary in over 50% of patients with hypertension. This permits the addition of primary actions of drugs while minimizing the homoeostatic compensations that limit the fall in pressure. Another advantage is that combination therapy causes fewer side effects as lower doses can be used.

12.3 Recommendations

12.3.1 *Policy and management*

1. A comprehensive strategy to prevent the complications associated with high blood pressure should make provision for both:

    (a) early identification and effective management of individuals with hypertension; and

    (b) prevention of hypertension by measures aimed at reducing the blood pressure levels in the population as a whole.

2. Arterial blood pressure should be measured (by the standard methods described in this report) in every individual seeking health care, in order to identify those who may require observation and treatment.

3. Before a person is labelled as hypertensive, raised blood pressure values should be confirmed by repeated measurements over a period of several weeks or months as blood pressure is quite variable.

4. In patients with borderline and mild hypertension, the level of blood pressure should be established by repeated measurements over several weeks or months before it is decided whether drug treatment is required. In patients with more severe hypertension, drug treatment should be instituted more rapidly and vigorously (see section 9.5).

5. In over 95% of cases of hypertension in adults, no specific cause can be identified (essential hypertension). Patients in whom a specific cause of hypertension is identified (secondary hypertension) require specific management (see section 9.5).

6. For patients with incipient diabetic nephropathy, treatment should be initiated at blood pressure values as low as SBP/DBP 130/85 mmHg (17.3/11.3 kPa).

7. In all cases, treatment should aim to achieve SBP/DBP levels of the order of 120–130/80 mmHg (16.0–17.3/10.7 kPa) in young and middle-aged patients, and below 140/90 mmHg (18.7/12.0 kPa) in the elderly.

8. The decision to treat should be based not only on the diastolic and systolic blood pressures but on an assessment of the total cardiovascular risk in the individual patient. The threshold for the initiation of drug treatment should be reduced as the total cardiovascular risk increases.

9. Lifestyle measures should be instituted in all patients with raised total cardiovascular risk, ranging from the normotensive through to those with moderate to severe hypertension. In some individuals with borderline and mild hypertension these measures may obviate the need for drug treatment. The measures which have been shown to lower blood pressure include weight restriction, reduction of alcohol intake, increased physical activity and moderation of dietary sodium.

10. Recommended first-line drugs for the treatment of hypertension are diuretics, β-blockers, ACE inhibitors, calcium antagonists and α-blockers. Other classes of drugs may be used in certain situations, for example during pregnancy and in low-income populations.

11. The choice of antihypertensive drugs should take into account socioeconomic factors that determine availability in different countries or regions. The choice should be largely determined by the characteristics of the individual patient, particularly by the level of risk for cardiovascular disease, the presence of target organ damage, the occurrence of side effects and coexisting disorders.

12. Effective two-way communication between the physician and the patient is critically important in the management of a chronic, life-long condition such as hypertension. It is essential that undergraduate and postgraduate educational programmes for physicians and other health professionals place a markedly increased emphasis on the acquisition of communication and counselling skills.

13. Since lifestyle measures (diet, exercise and reduced alcohol consumption) have been shown to be effective in reducing blood pressure levels in hypertensive individuals as well as in populations, they need to be promoted in communities as well as in clinical practice. The food industry should be encouraged to manufacture and market products with a low salt and fat content. Labelling of food products with their constituents would enable the consumer to exercise healthy choices.

14. Effective education programmes for the public, health professionals and patients should be developed to increase awareness of the causes and consequences of high blood pressure as well as methods for its prevention and control.

15. In developing countries, where major epidemics of cardiovascular disease are projected to occur or accelerate, the prevention of hypertension through population-based measures to improve lifestyle is strongly recommended.

16. The population and individual approaches to the prevention and control of hypertension are complementary and synergistic; both need to be incorporated into national control programmes for high blood pressure. Such programmes should correspond to the needs and resources of individual countries. These programmes should be built into all levels of health care, especially primary health care.

17. National hypertension societies and leagues should be encouraged to work in concert with national health authorities in the planning and implementation of national hypertension control programmes. These programmes should be guided by the contents of this report.

18. Health policy must include measures to promote blood pressure control through lifestyle measures, effective but inexpensive drug therapy and comprehensive community health education. This must be viewed in the context of an integrated approach to health promotion and disease prevention.

19. The cost-effectiveness of hypertension control should be analysed by programme managers. Systematic analyses of cost-effectiveness should be applied to all components of the individual patient approach and the population approach for the control of hyper-tension. This is critically important since it will permit all countries to select those strategies that maximize health benefits while containing costs at levels appropriate for the available resources.

20. In addition to cost–effectiveness, the methods and outcomes of hypertension control must be scientifically evaluated. Feedback from such studies will enable control programmes to be modified in order to make the most effective use of human and economic resources. Recommended approaches include: monitoring incidence rates of coronary events and stroke; surveys of prevalence, awareness and effectiveness of control; medical audit of case management practices; monitoring patients' perceptions of treatment; assessment of knowledge and attitudes of physicians; and drug utilization and food consumption patterns and trends.

12.3.2 *Research*

1. To provide the basis for appropriate public health interventions, epidemiological estimates of the prevalence of hypertension and the levels of risk factors leading to high blood pressure (or augmenting the risk of its complications) need to be obtained in all countries.

2. Several aspects of hypertension-related organ damage require better understanding:

   (a) although left ventricular hypertrophy is rightly considered an independent risk factor, it needs to be determined whether its risk declines with treatment-induced regression of hypertrophy;

   (b) the prevalence and clinical importance of reduced coronary reserve caused by coronary artery disease associated with hypertension should be better established, and trials carried out to determine whether it can be reversed;

   (c) although prevention of stroke by antihypertensive therapy has been very successful, more research is required to evaluate the effectiveness of antihypertensive therapy in preventing various types of stroke and recurrent stroke, and in affecting the development of vascular dementia;

   (d) as hypertension appears to remain a leading cause of kidney disease in spite of effective antihypertensive treatment, more research should be encouraged to clarify this paradox; the significance of microalbuminuria as an early marker of renal damage in hypertension should also be clarified.

3. Properly designed prospective studies are desirable to clarify the clinically important issue of "isolated clinic hypertension".

4. More research efforts should be concentrated on studying the mechanisms of hypertensive disease in pregnancy to facilitate prevention and develop suitable treatment.

5. Research into the genetic basis of hypertension should be encouraged. The information gained from specific genes and positional cloning

may identify new genetic polymorphisms that possibly influence blood pressure levels, cardiovascular risk and response to therapy. The findings of this research have the potential to improve the quality and methods of decision-making in the management and prevention of hypertension.

6. Since long-term and large clinical trials of antihypertensive treatment have not yet clearly demonstrated sex differences in response and outcomes, further study is warranted to determine whether a different management approach is needed in women than in men.

7. The Expert Committee recommends that the potential promised by medical information and computer technology be harnessed to assist physicians and health professionals to control hypertension and associated risk factors for cardiovascular disease in individual patients and in populations. The use of these techniques to assist in accessing the ever-growing mass of data should be evaluated. Sophisticated informatics programmes should also be developed to facilitate the assessment of total cardiovascular risk and to improve the quality of decision-making in hypertension control in both the individual patient and the community as a whole.

Acknowledgements

This report would be incomplete without an expression of gratitude to the following WHO staff members for their contribution to the success of this meeting:

Dr A. Alwan, Regional Adviser, Noncommunicable Diseases, WHO Regional Office for the Eastern Mediterranean, Alexandria, Egypt; Dr D. E. Barmes, Associate Director, Division of Noncommunicable Diseases, WHO, Geneva, Switzerland; Dr V. Boulyjenkov, Hereditary Diseases Programme, WHO, Geneva, Switzerland; Dr R. Buzina, Nutrition, WHO, Geneva, Switzerland; Dr M.R. Couper, Division of Drug Management and Policies, WHO, Geneva, Switzerland; Dr R. J. Guidotti, Medical Officer, Maternal Health and Safe Motherhood, WHO, Geneva, Switzerland; Dr H. V. Hogerzeil, Action Programme on Essential Drugs, WHO, Geneva, Switzerland; Dr N. Khaltaev, Acting Chief, Diabetes and Other Noncommunicable Diseases, WHO, Geneva, Switzerland; Dr I. Martin, Medical Officer, Cardiovascular Diseases, WHO, Geneva, Switzerland; Dr P. Nordet, Medical Officer, Cardiovascular Diseases, WHO, Geneva, Switzerland; Dr T. Ogada, Regional Officer, Noncommunicable Diseases, WHO Regional Office for Africa, Brazzaville, Congo; Mr T. M. Prentice, Information and Media Support, WHO, Geneva, Switzerland; Dr E. Pupulin, Acting Chief, Health of the Elderly, WHO, Geneva, Switzerland; Dr A. Shatchkute, Regional Adviser, Chronic Diseases, WHO Regional Office for Europe, Copenhagen, Denmark; Dr A. E. Wasunna, Clinical Technology, WHO, Geneva, Switzerland; and Dr Yu Sen-Hai, Health Education and Health Promotion, WHO, Geneva, Switzerland.

References

1. *Hypertension and coronary heart disease: classification and criteria for epidemiological studies. First Report of the Expert Committee on Cardiovascular Diseases and Hypertension.* Geneva, World Health Organization, 1959 (WHO Technical Report Series, No. 168).

2. *Arterial hypertension and ischaemic heart disease: preventive aspects. Report of a WHO Expert Committee.* Geneva, World Health Organization, 1962 (WHO Technical Report Series, No. 231).

3. *Arterial hypertension. Report of a WHO Expert Committee.* Geneva, World Health Organization, 1978 (WHO Technical Report Series, No. 628).

4. Pickering GW. *The nature of essential hypertension.* London, Churchill, 1961.

5. MacMahon S et al. Blood pressure, stroke and coronary heart disease. Part 1. Prolonged differences in blood pressure: prospective observational studies corrected for the regression dilution bias. *Lancet*, 1990, **335**:765-774.

6. Evans VG, Rose GA. Hypertension. *British medical bulletin,* 1971, **27**:32-42.

7. Kannel WB, Dawber TR, McGee DL. Perspectives on systolic hypertension: the Framingham Study. *Circulation*, 1986, **61**:1179-1182.

8. MRC Working Party on Mild to Moderate Hypertension. The MRC Mild Hypertension Trial: some subgroup results. In: Strasser T, Ganten D, eds. *Mild hypertension: from drug trials to practice.* New York, Raven Press, 1987:9-20.

9. Collins R et al. Blood pressure, stroke and coronary heart disease. Part 2. Short-term reductions in blood pressure: overview of randomized drug trials in their epidemiological context. *Lancet*, 1990, **335**:827-838.

10. SHEP Cooperative Research Group. Prevention of stroke by antihypertensive drug treatment in older persons with isolated systolic hypertension. *Journal of the American Medical Association,* 1991, **265**:3255-3264.

11. MRC Working Party. Medical Research Council trial of treatment of hypertension in older adults: principal results. *British medical journal,* 1992, **304**:405-412.

12. 1993 guidelines for the management of mild hypertension: memorandum from a WHO/ISH meeting. *Bulletin of the World Health Organization,* 1993, **71**:503-517.

13. Joint National Committee on Detection, Evaluation, and Treatment of High Blood Pressure. The fifth report of the Joint National Committee on Detection, Evaluation, and Treatment of High Blood Pressure (JNC V). *Archives of internal medicine,* 1993, **153**:154-183.

14. Amery A et al. Mortality and morbidity results from the European Working Party on High Blood Pressure in the Elderly trial. *Lancet*, 1985, i:1349-1354.

15. Dahlöf B et al. Morbidity and mortality in the Swedish Trial in Old Patients with Hypertension (STOP-Hypertension). *Lancet*, 1991, **338**:1281-1285.

16. MRC Working Party. Stroke and coronary heart disease in mild hypertension: risk factors and the value of treatment. *British medical journal*, 1988, **296**: 1565-1570.

17. Mancia G. Ambulatory blood pressure monitoring: research and clinical applications. *Journal of hypertension*, 1990, 8 (Suppl 7):S1-S13.

18. **Sega G et al.** Ambulatory and home blood pressure normality: the Pamela Study. *Journal of cardiovascular pharmacology,* 1994, **23** (Suppl.5):S12-S15.

19. **Mancia G et al.** Alerting reaction and rise in blood pressure during measurement by physician and nurse. *Hypertension,* 1987, **9**:209-215.

20. **Julius S et al.** White coat hypertension: a follow-up. *Clinical experimental hypertension,* 1992, **A14**:45-53.

21. **Stamler J, Stamler R, Neaton JD.** Blood pressure, systolic and diastolic, and cardiovascular risks: US population data. *Archives of internal medicine,* 1993, **153**:598-615.

22. **Kannel WB, Belanger AJ.** Epidemiology of heart failure. *American heart journal,* 1991, **121**:951-957.

23. **Whelton PK.** Epidemiology of hypertension. *Lancet,* 1994, **344**:101-106.

24. **Strasser T.** Equal blood pressure levels carry different risks in different risk factor combinations. *Journal of human hypertension,* 1992, **6**:261-264.

25. **Carvalho JJM et al.** Blood pressure in four remote populations in INTERSALT study. *Hypertension,* 1989, **14**:238-246.

26. **Alwan AAS.** Cardiovascular diseases in the Eastern Mediterranean Region. *World health statistics quarterly,* 1993, **46**(2):97-100.

27. **Reddy KS.** Cardiovascular diseases in India. *World health statistics quarterly,* 1993, **46**(2):101-107.

28. **Hungerbuhler P, Bovet P, Shamlaye C.** The cardiovascular disease situation in Seychelles. *World health statistics quarterly,* 1993, **46**(2):108-112.

29. **Yao Chonghua, Wu Zhaosu, Wu Yingkai.** The changing pattern of cardio-vascular disease in China. *World health statistics quarterly,* 1993, **46**(2):113-118.

30. **Boedhi-Darmojo R.** The pattern of cardiovascular disease in Indonesia. *World health statistics quarterly,* 1993, **46**(2):119-124.

31. **Muna WFT.** Cardiovascular disorders in Africa. *World health statistics quarterly,* 1993, **46**(2):125-133.

32. **Burt V et al.** Prevalence of hypertension in adult U.S. populations: results from the third National Health and Nutrition Examination Survey, 1988-91. *Hyper-tension,* 1995, **25**(3):305-313.

33. Geographical variation in the major risk factors of coronary heart disease in men and women aged 35-64 years. The WHO MONICA Project. *World health statistics quarterly,* 1988, **41**(3/4):115-140.

34. **Pickering G.** *High blood pressure.* London, Churchill, 1968.

35. **Julius S et al.** The association of borderline hypertension with target organ changes and higher coronary risk. Tecumseh Blood Pressure study. *Journal of the American Medical Association,* 1990, **264**:354-358.

36. **Williams RR et al.** Definition of genetic factors in hypertension: a search for major genes, polygenes, and homogeneous sub-types. *Journal of cardiovascular pharmacology,* 1988, **12**(Suppl. 3):S7-S20.

37. **Law CM et al.** Initiation of hypertension in utero and its amplification throughout life. *British medical journal,* 1993, **306**:24-27.

38. **MacMahon S et al.** Obesity and hypertension: epidemiological and clinical issues. *European heart journal,* 1987, **8**:57-70.

39. **Modan M, Kalkin H.** Hyperinsulinemia or increased sympathetic drive as links for obesity and hypertension. *Diabetes care,* 1991, **14**:470-487.

40. **Reaven GM.** Role of insulin resistance in human disease (1988 Banting lecture). *Diabetes,* 1988, **37**:1595-1607.

41. **Sharma AM.** Effects of nonpharmacological intervention on insulin sensitivity. *Journal of cardiovascular pharmacology,* 1992, **20**:S27-S34.

42. **Elliott P.** Observational studies of salt and blood pressure. *Hypertension,* 1991, **17**(Suppl. 1):103-108.

43. **Law MR, Frost CD, Wald NJ.** By how much does dietary salt reduction lower blood pressure? I: Analysis of observational data among populations. *British medical journal,* 1991, **302**:811-815.

44. **Stamler R.** Implications of the INTERSALT study. *Hypertension,* 1991, **17**(Suppl. 1):1017-1020.

45. **INTERSALT Cooperative Research Group.** INTERSALT: an international study of electrolyte excretion and blood pressure: results for 24-hour urinary sodium and potassium excretion. *British medical journal,* 1988, **297**:319-328.

46. **Yamori Y et al.** Gene environment interaction in hypertension, stroke and atherosclerosis in experimental models and supportive findings from a worldwide cross-sectional epidemiological survey: a WHO-CARDIAC Study. *Clinical experimental pharmacology, physiology supplement,* 1992, **20**:43-52.

47. **Pearce KA, Furberg CD.** The primary prevention of hypertension. *Cardiovascular risk factors,* 1994, **4**:147-153.

48. **Paffenbarger RS et al.** Physical activity and incidence of hypertension in college alumni. *American journal of epidemiology,* 1983, **117**:245-257.

49. **Esler M et al.** Overflow of catecholamine neurotransmitters to the circulation: source, fate and function. *Physiological reviews,* 1990, **70**:963-986.

50. **Anderson EA et al.** Elevated sympathetic nerve activity in borderline hypertensive humans. *Hypertension,* 1989, **14**:177-183.

51. **Mancia G et al.** Evaluating sympathetic activity in human hypertension. *Journal of hypertension,* 1993, **11**(Suppl. 5):S13-S19.

52. **Zanchetti A, Mancia G.** Cardiovascular reflexes and hypertension. *Hypertension,* 1991, **18**(Suppl. III):13-21.

53. **Cowley AW, Roman RJ.** The pressure diuresis mechanism in normal and hypertensive states. In: Zanchetti A, Tarazi RC, eds. *Pathophysiology of hypertension: regulatory mechanisms.* Amsterdam, Elsevier, 1986:295-314 (Handbook of hypertension, Vol. 8).

54. **Waeber B, Nussberger J, Brunner HR.** The renin angiotensin system: role in experimental and human hypertension. In: Zanchetti A, Tarazi RC, eds. *Pathophysiology of hypertension: regulatory mechanisms.* Amsterdam, Elsevier, 1986:489-519 (Handbook of hypertension, Vol. 8).

55. **Folkow B.** Current thinking in hypertension – peripheral vasculature. *Blood pressure,* 1992, **1**(Suppl.l):7-10.

56. **Koren MJ et al.** Relation of left ventricular mass and geometry to morbidity and mortality in uncomplicated essential hypertension. *Annals of internal medicine,* 1991, **114**:345-352.

57. **Korner PI.** Some thoughts on pathogenesis, therapy and prevention of hypertension. *Blood pressure,* 1994, **3**:7-17.

58. **Lüscher TF et al.** Interactions between platelets and the vessel wall. Role of endothelium-derived vasoactive substances. In: Laragh JH, Brenner BM, eds. *Hypertension: pathophysiology, diagnosis and management.* New York, Raven Press, 1990:637-648.

59. **Liu LS et al.** Secondary hypertension in the community and among hospitalized hypertensive patients. *Acta academiae medicinae sinicae,* 1980, **2**:236-240.

60. **Swales J, ed.** *Textbook of hypertension.* Oxford, Blackwell, 1994.

61. **Zanchetti A, Sleight P, Birkenhäger WH.** Evaluation of organ damage in hypertension. *Journal of hypertension,* 1993, **11**:875-882.

62. **Kannel WB.** Left ventricular hypertrophy as a risk factor: the Framingham experience. *Journal of hypertension,* 1991, **9**(Suppl. 2):S3-S9.

63. **Levy D et al.** Prognostic implications of echocardiographically determined left ventricular mass in the Framingham Heart Study. *New England journal of medicine,* 1990, **332**:1561-1566.

64. **Koren MJ et al.** Relation of left ventricular mass and geometry to morbidity and mortality in uncomplicated essential hypertension. *Annals of internal medicine,* 1991, **114**:345-352.

65. **Devereux RB.** Left ventricular diastolic dysfunction: early diastolic relaxation and late diastolic compliance. *Journal of the American College of Cardiology,* 1989, **13**:337-339.

66. **Strauer BE.** *The hypertensive heart,* 3rd ed. Berlin, Springer-Verlag, 1991.

67. **Yussuf S, Thom T, Abbott RD.** Changes in hypertension treatment and in congestive heart failure mortality in the United States. *Hypertension,* 1989, **13**(Suppl. 1):174-179.

68. **Birkenhäger WH, De Leeuw PW.** Hypertension, antihypertensive treatment, and kidney. *Blood pressure,* 1992, **1**:201-207.

69. **Kannel WB et al.** The prognostic significance of proteinuria: the Framingham Study. *American heart journal,* 1984, **108**:1347-1352.

70. **Ruilope LM.** Proteinuria and renal function. *Blood pressure,* 1993, **2**(Suppl.1): 55-58.

71. **Rosansky SJ et al.** The association of blood pressure levels and change in renal functions in hypertensive and nonhypertensive subjects. *Archives of internal medicine,* 1990, **150**:2073-2074.

72. **Gross F et al.** *Management of arterial hypertension: a practical guide for the physician and allied health workers.* Geneva, World Health Organization, 1984.

73. **Task Force on Blood Pressure Control in Children.** Report of the Second Task Force on Blood Pressure Control in Children. *Pediatrics,* 1987, **79**:1-25.

74. **Layde PM, Beral V, Kay CR.** Further analyses of mortality in oral contraceptive users. Royal College of General Practitioners' Oral Contraception Study. *Lancet,* 1981, i:541-546.

75. **Wren BG, Routledge DA.** Blood pressure changes: oestrogens in climacteric women. *Medical journal of Australia,* 1981, **2**:528-531.

76. **Kincaid-Smith P.** Hypertension in pregnancy. *Blood pressure,* 1994, **3**:18-23.

77. **Davey DA, McGilliveat I.** A classification of the hypertensive disorders of pregnancy. *Clinical experimental hypertension,* 1986, **A5**:97-133.

78. **Kannel WB.** Hypertension and the risk of cardiovascular disease. In: Laragh JH, Brenner BM, eds. *Hypertension: pathophysiology, diagnosis and management.* New York, Raven Press, 1990:101-117.

79. **Epstein M, Sowers JR.** Diabetes mellitus and hypertension. *Hypertension,* 1992, **19**:403-418.

80. **Rose G.** Sick individuals and sick populations. *International journal of epidemiology,* 1985, **14**:32-38.

81. **National High Blood Pressure Education Working Group.** Report on primary prevention of hypertension. *Archives of internal medicine,* 1993, **153**:186-208.

82. **Stevens VJ et al.** Weight loss intervention in phase 1 of the Trials of Hypertension Prevention. *Archives of internal medicine,* 1993, **153**:849-858.

83. **The Trials of Hypertension Prevention Collaborative Research Group.** The effects of nonpharmacologic interventions on blood pressure of persons with high normal levels: results of the trials of hypertension prevention. Phase I. *Journal of the American Medical Association,* 1992, **267**:1213-1220.

84. **Puddey IB, Beilin LJ, Vandongen R.** Regular alcohol use raises blood pressure in treated hypertensive subjects. *Lancet,* 1987, i:647-651.

85. **Puddey IB et al.** Effects of alcohol and caloric restriction on blood pressure and serum lipids in overweight men. *Hypertension,* 1992, **20**:533-541.

86. **Paffenbarger RS Jr et al.** Physical activity and hypertension. An epidemiological view. *Annals of medicine,* 1991, **23**:319-327.

87. **Arakawa K.** Hypertension and exercise. *Clinical experimental hypertension,* 1993, **15**:1171-1179.

88. **Arroll B, Beaglehole R.** Does physical activity lower blood pressure? A critical review of clinical trials. *Journal of clinical epidemiology,* 1992, **45**:439-447.

89. **Frost CD, Law MR, Wald NJ.** By how much does dietary salt reduction lower blood pressure? II: Analysis of observational data within populations. *British medical journal,* 1991, **302**:815-818.

90. **Cutler JA et al.** An overview of randomized trials of sodium restriction and blood pressure. *Hypertension,* 1991, **17**(Suppl.1):27-33.

91. **Law MR, Frost CD, Wald NJ.** By how much does dietary salt reduction lower blood pressure? III: Analysis of data from trials of salt reduction. *British medical journal,* 1991, **302**:819-824.

92. **Medical Research Council Working Party.** MRC trial of treatment of mild hypertension: principal results. *British medical journal,* 1985, **291**:97-104.

93. **Manson JE et al.** The primary prevention of myocardial infarction. *New England journal of medicine,* 1992, **326**:1406-1416.

94. Stamler R, Stamler J, Gosch FC. Primary prevention of hypertension by nutritional-hygienic means: final results of randomized controlled trial. *Journal of the American Medical Association,* 1989, 262:1801-1807.

95. Hypertension Prevention Trial Research Group. The hypertension prevention trial. Three year effects of dietary changes on blood pressure. *Archives of internal medicine,* 1990, 150:153-162.

96. Zanchetti A. Goals of antihypertensive treatment: prevention of cardiovascular events and prevention of organ damage. *Blood pressure,* 1992, 1:205-211.

97. Lithell H. Insulin resistance and cardiovascular drugs. *Clinical experimental hypertension,* 1992, A14:151-162.

98. Yusuf S et al. Beta blockade during and after myocardial infarction: An overview of the randomized trials. *Progress in cardiovascular diseases,* 1985, XXVII: 335-371.

99. Kreft-Jais C, Plouin PF, Tchobroutsky C. Angiotensin converting enzyme inhibition with captopril in human pregnancy. *Journal of hypertension,* 1987, 5(Suppl.5):S553-S554.

100. The SOLVD Investigators. Effect of enalapril on mortality and the development of heart failure in asymptomatic patients with reduced left ventricular ejection fraction. *New England journal of medicine,* 1992, 327:685-691.

101. Pfeffer MA et al. Effects of captopril on mortality and morbidity in patients with left ventricular dysfunction after myocardial infarction. Results of the survival and ventricular enlargement trials. *New England journal of medicine,* 1992, 327:669-677.

102. Dahlöf B, Pennert K and Hansson L. Reversal of left ventricular hypertrophy in hypertensive patients: a meta-analysis of 109 treatment studies. *American journal of hypertension,* 1992, 5:95-110.

103. Lewis EJ et al. The effect of angiotensin-converting-enzyme inhibition on diabetic nephropathy. *New England journal of medicine,* 1993, 329(20): 1456-1462.

104. Chalmers JP. The place of combination therapy in the treatment of hypertension in 1993. *Clinical experimental hypertension,* 1993, 15(6):1299-1313.

105. Wassertheil-Smoller S et al. The Trial of Antihypertensive Interventions and Management (TAIM) Study. Final results with regard to blood pressure, cardiovascular risk and quality of life. *American journal of hypertension,* 1992, 5(1):37-44.

106. Siani A et al. Increasing the dietary potassium intake reduces the need for anti-hypertensive medication. *Annals of internal medicine,* 1991, 115:753-759.

107. Beard TC et al. Randomised controlled trial of a no-added-sodium diet for mild hypertension. *Lancet,* 1982, ii:455-458.

108. Neaton JD et al. Treatment of Mild Hypertension Study. Final results. *Journal of the American Medical Association,* 1993, 270(6):713-724.

109. Cutler JA. Combinations of lifestyle modification and drug treatment in management of mild-moderate hypertension: a review of randomised clinical trials. *Clinical experimental hypertension,* 1993, 15(6):1193-1204.

110. Grueninger UJ, Goldstein MG, Diffy FD. A conceptual framework for interactive patient education in practice and clinic settings. *Journal of human hypertension,* 1990, 4(Suppl.1):21-31.

111. Weinstein MC, Stason WB. *Hypertension: a policy perspective.* Boston, Harvard University Press, 1976.

112. Fletcher A. Pressure to treat and pressure to cost: a review of cost-effectiveness analysis. *Journal of hypertension,* 1991, **9**:193-198.

113. Johannesson M, Jönsson B. A review of cost-effectiveness analyses of hypertension treatment. *Pharmaco-Economics,* 1992, **1**:250-264.

114. Johannesson M et al. The cost-effectiveness of treating hypertension in elderly people – an analysis of the Swedish Trial in Old Patients with Hypertension (STOP Hypertension). *Journal of internal medicine,* 1993, **234**:317-323.

115. Ménard J, Cornu P, Day M. Cost of hypertension treatment and the price of health. *Journal of human hypertension,* 1992, **6**:447-458.

116. *The use of essential drugs. Sixth report of the WHO Expert Committee.* Geneva, World Health Organization, 1995 (WHO Technical Report Series, No. 850).

117. Ambrosio GB et al. Effects of interventions on community awareness and treatment of hypertension: results of a WHO study. *Bulletin of the World Health Organization,* 1988, **66**(1):107-113.

118. Strasser T, Wilhelmsen L, eds. Assessing hypertension control and management. *Hypertension Management Audit Project: a WHO/WHL study.* Copenhagen, World Health Organization, 1993 (WHO Regional Publications, European Series No. 47).

119. Wilhelmsen L, Strasser T. WHO/WHL Hypertension Management Audit Project. *Journal of human hypertension,* 1993, **7**:257-263.

120. Rocella EJ, Lenfant C. Considerations regarding the cost and effectiveness of public and patient education programmes. *Journal of human hypertension,* 1992, **6**:463-467.

World Health Organization Technical Report Series

---

* Prices in developing countries are 70% of those listed here.